WALKING MY TALK
TO SUCCESS

How to **WIN** *in life*

First Edition

Editing Services by Caitlin Freeman of Get Bookified
Book Cover, Typesetting and Layout Design Copyright © 2022 Maja Creative
Art Direction by Maja Wolnik of Maja Creative
Graphic Design by Monika Brzeczek of Maja Creative
Cover Photography by Antoinette Dakota-Rainer

ISBN PRINT: 978-0-6454260-0-7
ISBN EBOOK: 978-0-6454260-1-4

Published by OJTS Personal Coaching

TABLE OF CONTENTS

CHAPTER

01

UNDERSTANDING SEVERE LANGUAGE DISORDER

Having a learning disability can lead to many challenges in life. One of the most difficult times is during school. When kids have learning differences, it can put immense pressure on them and their families, especially when they don't have extra support from their teachers. I was in my own world throughout my school years. My teachers didn't know what to do with me at first. I was not able to speak until I was four years old, and even after I started talking, I had difficulty engaging in conversations. I had a severe stutter, and I struggled to find the words that I wanted to say. Eventually, I was diagnosed with Severe Language Disorder.

My parents realised that something was wrong when I was a toddler. Other children had started speaking simple words, but I remained persistently mute. My mother later told me about a conversation that she had with my father about her concerns.

'Boris, shouldn't Oliver have started talking by now?'

'Maybe he is just taking his time', my father replied. 'He's only one year old, so we can just wait and see.'

'I guess so', said my mother. 'I'm just afraid that there is something wrong with him. I'm worried that he might not live a normal life.'

Two years passed, and I was still yet to say my first word. This raised more concerns with my parents, and they decided that it was time to do something. My mum looked into several paediatric speech pathologists for me, and eventually she found a doctor she liked. I remember her name was Dr. Kelly, and she had an office in the city. My dad agreed to take me in, and they booked an appointment with her.

My parents and I arrived at the speech pathologist's office at the Royal Children's Hospital. The doctor put me through several aptitude tests to see if my intelligence had been affected. She wanted to rule out mental retardation before she could give me a formal diagnosis. When the results came back, she told my parents that my intelligence was normal. I was just slow to speak. She diagnosed me with a language delay due to Severe Language Disorder, and she explained to my parents that I would start speaking in my own time. My mum was relieved to have a name for my condition, but she was still concerned that my differences would affect the quality of my life.

As I reached the age of four, I began saying my first words. My parents were both hugely relieved that I would not spend my life non-verbal. My mum phoned her mother to announce the good news. Her excitement was tempered with the realisation that I still had a tough road ahead of me. Dr. Kelly, my speech pathologist, had warned her that school would likely be difficult. I had a lot of learning to do to catch up with my peers. Nevertheless, my mum was determined to give me as close to a normal life as possible.

I began school at the age of five. My parents sent me to the Knox School, which was a private school near our house. My parents tried to explain what school would be like, but nothing they said could have prepared me for the experience of that first day. My mum took me to school and introduced me to my teacher, Mrs. Robinson. I was fine until my mum said goodbye. As soon as she left the classroom, I broke down and started crying. This was an overwhelming new experience for me. I told her, 'I don't want to be here. I want to go home.' Mrs. Robinson was sympathetic, but she didn't know how to comfort me. 'Come on, Oliver', she told me. 'Let's sit you down here at this table. I promise you will have fun.' She tried to engage me in an activity, but I continued to cry up until recess, where I finally settled in. I played by myself during recess and lunch. I was an independent child, and I didn't have any particular interest in the other children. Besides, I wouldn't have known how to play with them even if I did.

My learning disability really began to show when I commenced grade one the following year. I was easily distractable, and my attention would drift from one thing to another. Sometimes I would sit on the floor and gaze up at the ceiling fans. Soon, I started falling behind in my schoolwork. My teacher, Mrs. Gannon, grew worried as my level slipped further and further below that of the other kids. After a few weeks, she brought my parents in for a conference. My mum and dad informed her of my diagnosis and explained that I had only started speaking two years before. The school didn't have many supports for children with learning delays. Mrs. Gannon knew that I would not be ready to advance to grade two at the end of the year. Her best advice was to recommend that I repeat grade one next year. She also arranged for a special aid teacher to help me for the rest of the year. She tried to reassure my parents that I wouldn't be the only child repeating a grade. 'Don't worry', she told them. 'I'm sure he will come across other kids who have repeated a year. Make sure to tell him that you're not disappointed in him; this is for his own good so he can get better in class.'

When my parents came home from the conference that afternoon, they told me that I would be repeating the first grade. I didn't understand what this would mean for me. I was too distracted to understand what was happening in my young life. When I came back to school the following day, I saw Mrs. Gannon leading another teacher over to my seat. 'Hi Oliver', said the woman. 'My name is Mrs. Thompson. I will be here to support you in class this year and next.' Mrs. Thompson was as good as her word. She helped me get up to speed in my subjects and made it possible for me to stay in school without slipping too far out of my age cohort. Looking back, I am so glad that I had this extra help. I know that I would have continued to struggle if I had been forced to learn independently.

The following year, I returned to my first-grade classroom and saw a sea of new faces staring at me. These students had all been in prep the year before, so I was now the oldest child in the class. Mrs. Gannon stood at the front of the classroom. She was my teacher once again. I chose a seat at the back of the class. As I sat down, Mrs. Gannon announced, 'Everyone, the young boy sitting on the back left is Oliver. He is repeating grade one. If you see another teacher sitting next to Oliver, they are here to support him.'

As I listened to Mrs. Gannon's announcement, I felt mortified and confused. Why did she have to single me out like that in front of the class? Didn't she know how cruel children can be to those they view as different? These younger kids were not going to treat me like I was older and wiser; they were going to treat me like a freak. I did not know how I was going to cope for the rest of the year.

Thank goodness I had my studies. As a consolation for repeating first grade, Mrs. Gannon allowed me to focus on my special interests in class.

'Oliver, you will need to come up with a presentation this year. The rest of the class is presenting on bicycles, like you did last year. So, this year, you get to pick a topic that you are interested in.'

'Okay, I want to do my topic based on planes', I replied.

'You certainly can if you like. Do you know much about planes, Oliver?'

'Yes! It's my favourite topic.'

Nothing excited me more as a child than travelling by air. The first time I remember flying was when I was five or six years old. I was nervous at first, but as the plane took off into the sky, I realised that this was exactly where I wanted to be. From then on, I would feel a thrill of excitement every time I waited at the gate, standing face to face with a 747-400.

My father's family is from Croatia, and we would fly there every year in July to visit my grandparents. My father is from Zadar, but my grandparents moved to the island of Iž when I was young. I loved my time there. The island is small, and everyone knows everyone else. My grandparents' house was only a five-minute walk from the beach, so every morning and afternoon I would spend hours playing in the water.

Croatia was a beautiful place to be a little kid. The only thing better than the visit was the plane ride over. I remember at one of our layovers in Singapore, the captain invited my brother Daniel and me into the flight deck. That felt really special and left a lasting impression on me. My parents would always ask for a window seat for me, and they would make sure that we were seated directly behind the wing so that I could watch the action during take-off and landing.

This passion helped me get through grade one for the second time. I began working on my assignment with assistance from Mrs. Thompson. Both Mrs. Gannon and Mrs. Thompson were impressed with my knowledge of aviation at such a young age, and they gave me good marks on my presentation.

> **I WAS NOT ABLE TO SPEAK UNTIL I WAS FOUR YEARS OLD, AND EVEN AFTER I STARTED TALKING, I HAD DIFFICULTY ENGAGING IN CONVERSATIONS. I HAD A SEVERE STUTTER, AND I STRUGGLED TO FIND THE WORDS THAT I WANTED TO SAY. EVENTUALLY, I WAS DIAGNOSED WITH SEVERE LANGUAGE DISORDER.**

By the end of the year, I achieved high enough marks to move up to grade two the following year. When I entered the second-grade classroom, my teacher, Mrs. McQuitty, informed the class that our homework load was going to increase. 'You will all need to start working harder this year', she announced in a stern voice. 'Each level you complete in school will become more challenging, so make sure that you pay attention in class and do your homework every day.' I didn't know how I was going to make it through this year. The school didn't provide me with an aid like they had in first grade, and I knew that I was going to struggle without the extra support.

Sure enough, I began to have trouble only a few weeks into second grade. Mrs. McQuitty pulled me aside one day to tell me that she was displeased with my progress.

'Oliver, you're not showing enough effort in school, and you are barely doing your homework. What is going on?'

'I'm not sure, Miss', I replied in a quiet voice as I struggled to find the answer.

'Well, you will need to work harder, or else you will risk failing grade two. Now, I am sure you don't want that to happen, do you?'

'Um, no Miss', I said. I was terrified of being left behind another grade. It was embarrassing enough being a year behind my age-mates. A two-year age gap would be mortifying.

As the year progressed, my academic skills slowly began to improve. I got better at taking the weekly tests in class, and I started completing my homework on time. I remember running down from the arts room one day and announcing to Mrs. McQuitty, 'Miss! Miss! I did my English homework last night!' I was so pleased that I had managed to finish my assignment.

Mrs. McQuitty bent down to my level and said, 'Oliver, I am delighted to hear that.'

I was relieved that she seemed happy with my progress; however, I was still concerned that I would be held back another year. I desperately wanted to move up to the next level. Then one day towards the end of school, Mrs. McQuitty announced to the class, 'Now, remember everyone that you have your afternoon with Mrs. Newton today. She will be your grade three teacher.' As we all made our way to the room next door, I let out a sigh of relief. It looked like I wouldn't have to repeat grade two after all.

When I began grade three the following year, my attention span started to improve, and I became more comfortable with my studies. At the first parent-teacher conference, my teacher Mrs. Newton told my parents that I was doing well in class despite my language delay. 'His weekly test results are almost perfect', she said. 'I can tell that he is a bright young man.' My mum was relieved. She told my teacher she was worried that my disability would continue to hold me back at school.

Throughout the year, my learning speed increased, and my grades continued to improve. Just as I was about to finish grade three, my parents called my brother and me to the family table. 'Oliver and Daniel, things are going to change for you next year', my mum told us. 'You won't be continuing on at the Knox School. It is costing us too much to keep you both there, so we are moving you to new schools', she explained. 'Oliver, I have enrolled you in Jells Park Primary School. Daniel, you will be going to Brentwood Secondary College.' I naturally felt upset about this decision. Looking back, however, I understand why my parents had to make this difficult decision.

Grade four began, and I was taken to Jells Park Primary School. I was hit with culture shock as I had transitioned from a strict private school to a more relaxed public school. On the first day, my teacher, Mr. Larrie, stood me up in front of the classroom. 'Everyone, this is Oliver. He is a new student from the Knox School. Please make him feel welcome.'

As I went to take my seat, a student waved at me. 'You can come and sit here with us if you like. I'm Sanjeevan.' I sat down and attempted to make conversation, but I felt awkward and uncomfortable. I was quiet and shy, and I spoke with a stutter. As much as I tried to blend in with the other kids, I knew that I would have difficulty making new friends.

As the year carried on, several of the students in my grade started bullying me for my language delay. The worst was a boy named Mark. He was taller than me with a perpetually aggressive look on his face. He didn't have many friends, but he still commanded respect. Every time he spoke, everyone had to listen to him, or he would lose his temper.

Mark started bullying me with verbal taunts. One time, I remember he walked up to me and sneered, 'Why isn't the baby talking?'

'I can talk. I just sometimes choose not to', I replied quietly.

'Did you just talk back at me? You better think twice about the way you're speaking to me!'

Mark's taunts soon turned physical. At lunch break, he grabbed me and started kicking me on the backside. He didn't let go until I was black and blue. After that, he would beat me up any chance he got. I would regularly come home from school with bruises.

Mark's physical abuse finally stopped when I began hanging out with Sanjeevan and his friends. They provided me with some degree of protection. I would play cricket with them during our breaks. I didn't know how to bowl properly, but Sanjeevan stepped in and showed me a few tips. 'You want to make sure that your arm is as straight as possible when you let go of the ball. Keep your head up and your eyes focused on the wickets.' I practiced the move over and over, and slowly I got better. During my final years of primary school, I was even given an opportunity to play cricket for the interschool competition.

The school year soon came to an end, and I started preparing to begin secondary school at Brentwood the next year. I felt excited about the transition, but I knew it was going to be challenging. I was right to be nervous. I struggled to fit in, and I found it difficult even to participate in conversations with my fellow students. The other kids saw me as a target, and they began bullying me nearly every day. My classmates would say things like, 'Hey Oliver, why don't you talk? You're just a big baby, aren't you?' When I tried to respond, they would say, 'Hey, who said you could talk back to us? You better keep your mouth shut unless you want us to beat you up!' The bullying soon turned violent, and I was once again going home black and blue.

I finally told my mum what was going on, and she arranged for me to switch to St. Francis Xavier College the following year. As the school year came to an end, I felt an immense sense of relief as I finished my final day at Brentwood. I couldn't bear the thought of being beaten up for even one more day. Never again would I have to tolerate kids hitting me, shoving me into lockers, and threatening to put me in the hospital. I used the summer holidays to unwind and prepare for new beginnings. An added bonus was that my new school was much closer to my house. It was a strange feeling not having to wake up for school at 5:30 in the morning. I left home at 7:30 a.m. and took the train to school, which was only an eight-minute ride.

Thankfully, the kids at St. Francis Xavier College were friendly, and they made me feel welcome. It was such a relief to get along with my classmates and not feel anxious about coming to school every day. The teachers at my new school were both kind and observant. They noticed that I was struggling with my language delay, and they recommended that I see a specialist. I went to a speech pathology centre in Hawthorn. The speech pathologist confirmed my diagnosis of Severe Language Disorder. He told my mum, 'This is not an uncommon disability. Essentially, Oliver can go on to live a normal life in certain regards. However, the reality is that Oliver won't be able to have a successful career due to his disability.' As a man who has now created a successful career for himself, I look back at this exchange and shudder. I didn't realise it at the time, but I was about to set out on a mission to prove this doctor's prognosis wrong.

NOTHING EXCITED ME MORE AS A CHILD THAN TRAVELLING BY AIR. THE FIRST TIME I REMEMBER FLYING WAS WHEN I WAS FIVE OR SIX YEARS OLD. I WAS NERVOUS AT FIRST, BUT AS THE PLANE TOOK OFF INTO THE SKY, I REALISED THAT THIS WAS EXACTLY WHERE I WANTED TO BE. FROM THEN ON, I WOULD FEEL A THRILL OF EXCITEMENT EVERY TIME I WAITED AT THE GATE, STANDING FACE TO FACE WITH A 747-400.

Growing up with a disability does not mean that a child cannot live a normal or successful life. If you are a parent and your child has been diagnosed with a learning disability, the best thing you can do is to support them throughout their school years. Be patient. Don't rush your child. If they are slow to talk, allow them to start speaking at their own time. Let them know that this is nothing for them to feel embarrassed about. I want you to recognise that there is help out there. You will find qualified specialists, but you will have to search for this support. It is essential to advocate for your child until they get the help that they need. Your dedication is the key ingredient that will set them up for success in life. As your child gets older, people will appreciate what they have gone through. Trust me when I tell you that it really does get better.

02

EXPERIENCING ROCK BOTTOM

At some point in our lives, most of us will experience anxiety and depression. This is not a pleasant journey for anyone to go through. There are ways that we can deal with these challenges, such as seeking help from a doctor, reaching out to family and friends, and working on our own mental health. Sadly, many who struggle with depression may not see any way out other than taking their own lives.

As my final term of year 11 commenced, the pressure of mounting schoolwork and the stress of upcoming exams started to become too much for me. Each night, I had more trouble sleeping, and my appetite slowly decreased. I began to worry about my health. Anxious thoughts of serious illness flooded my mind. People with cancer lose their appetites, don't they? After all, I knew someone once who had a brain tumour, and he lost his appetite. My anxiety kept spiralling upwards. One morning, I woke up feeling like there was a dark cloud hanging over me. All I felt was pure sadness and unworthiness. When I went to school that day, I decided to see the school psychologist, Mrs. Murphy, who had an appointment available that afternoon.

'Hi Oliver, please come on in', said Mrs. Murphy as I opened the door. 'So, what brings you here today?'

'I-I guess I've been under a lot of stress', I stammered. 'I haven't been feeling like myself. I'm not sleeping well, and I've pretty much lost my appetite.'

Mrs. Murphy took out a pen and paper. 'Okay, let's go into that', she replied. 'Do you feel that the stress may be caused by upcoming exams?'

'It may be that', I said. 'I also am having constant thoughts that I have a tumour or leukaemia. I know someone who had a brain tumour. He lost his appetite, too.'

'You know, you're not the only one who has concerns over getting a serious illness. Sometimes we get a headache, and we think that it's something concerning. Then we realise that it's just a headache. If you're still concerned, you can visit your doctor. Meanwhile, I can help you manage your stress.'

We carried on the conversation for the rest of the afternoon, addressing my wellbeing. 'Now, do you need to take tomorrow off?' asked Mrs. Murphy.

'No', I shook my head. 'I think I'll be okay coming to school.'

The next morning, I woke up feeling like the black cloud hanging over me had grown even bigger. I had barely slept, and my appetite was nonexistent. I practically had to force myself to eat. I had a small bowl of fruit salad before leaving, as the thought of having a full breakfast made me want to vomit. I made my way to school, and I knew straightaway that something was not right.

As I walked to my first class, my thoughts began racing. I started questioning whether it was worth it to go on living.

My P.E. teacher, Mrs. Arangurin, caught me in the hallway. She could tell that something was wrong. 'Oliver is everything okay?' she asked me, a worried look furrowing her brows.

'I'm not sure, to be honest', I replied, trying to blink back tears. 'I haven't been feeling like myself lately. I'm not happy at all, and I'm just struggling to come to school every day.'

'Oh. Well, maybe it's worth it for you to see a therapist or a counsellor that you can talk to', she told me. She looked concerned, but she couldn't stay to chat for long. She had to rush to teach her next class.

I made my way to my Religious Education class and felt no change in my mental wellbeing. As I approached the classroom door, I saw my friend Josh standing outside, waiting for the period to start. He looked up, and as soon as he saw me, his eyes widened. 'Hey, Oli! Everything okay?'

I must have looked down in the dumps. I tried to smile, but I could barely make my mouth move. 'Hey, Josh. I don't know', I replied, shaking my head. 'I just haven't been feeling like myself over the last week or so.'

'Sorry to hear that, mate. What's going on?' asked Josh.

'I've been feeling really sad, and I just haven't been able to cheer myself up.'

'That's tough. Have you talked to someone about it? There are people here that you can talk to.'

'Yeah, but I don't feel that they really care that much. Probably because I was bullied quite badly at my last school.'

'Well, there are people here that care about you, you know. We're here for you, mate', said Josh as we walked into class.

After being bullied for so many years, I found it difficult to digest what Josh had just said. I knew that many of the students at my year level did not appreciate me for who I was due to my lack of confidence; however, there was a small handful that did care about my wellbeing. As much as I wanted to believe Josh's words, I still felt that I had no one to turn to. As I made my way back to my house at the end of the school day, the dark cloud over my head grew even larger. I felt that I had reached a breaking point. The thought of continuing on became too much for me. Something within me urged me to end my own life.

MY ANXIETY KEPT SPIRALLING UPWARDS. ONE MORNING, I WOKE UP FEELING LIKE THERE WAS A DARK CLOUD HANGING OVER ME. ALL I FELT WAS PURE SADNESS AND UNWORTHINESS

That afternoon when I arrived home, I decided to talk to my father about the heavy thoughts I was having. 'Dad, I don't think I want to live anymore', I said in desperation.

'What? Why?' asked dad. 'Come here and sit down.'

I sat down beside him, with my anxiety growing even stronger.

'Now, Oliver, tell me, why are you thinking like that?'

'I don't know. Everything is just becoming too much for me.'

'Do you want to see if Dr. Oechsle is available?' asked dad.

'Yes, I'll call him now', I nodded. I phoned the Casey Medical Centre, hoping to get an appointment with my doctor. 'Hi, I was wondering if I could speak to Dr. Oechsle, if he is available?' I asked the clerk. 'It is pretty serious', I added.

'Okay, let me see if I can get a hold of him for you', the clerk replied.

I waited on hold, praying that I would be able to get through.

After a few minutes, Dr. Oechsle answered the phone. 'Hello, Oliver.

How are you doing?'

'Not too great, actually. I'm having thoughts of ending my own life', I replied.

'Oh really?' said Dr. Oechsle, sounding concerned. 'Do you want to pop into the office this afternoon?'

'Yes, please. Whenever you have time available.'

'I will be available in the next fifteen minutes, so I'm happy for you to come down as soon as you can.'

My dad and I got in the car, and we went straight to the medical centre for my emergency appointment. We arrived at the doctor's office after a ten-minute drive, and I sat in the waiting area, hoping to be called into the office soon.

'Oliver, come on in', said Dr. Oechsle as he stepped out into the waiting room. I got up and walked straight into his office, slumping into a seat next to his desk.

'Your call got me concerned', said Dr. Oechsle. 'Talk to me about what's going on.'

'I don't know exactly', I said, staring at my hands. 'It's been happening for at least the last few weeks. I've been feeling a lot of stress and anxiety. It's gotten progressively worse over the last few days. I haven't been sleeping properly, and I've lost my appetite.'

'Is there anything in particular that's causing this stress? Is it from school, do you think?'

'I'm not sure if school is a contributor, but I've been having thoughts popping up in my head telling me that I have leukaemia or a tumour.'

'Okay. What has caused that sort of concern?'

'Well, I have a friend who suffered a brain tumour', I replied. 'The symptoms he had at the beginning are a lot like what I've been experiencing recently. He's okay now, but the ordeal he went through really scared me. I can feel myself spiralling into this hole that I can't seem to get out of.'

'Well, Oliver, we can run some tests to see if there is anything wrong, but I want to reassure you that cancer isn't contagious, and brain tumours are much rarer than you think', said Dr. Oechsle. 'Just because someone you know had a tumour doesn't mean you will have it.'

'I've been telling myself that', I nodded. 'Still, every time I try to reason with myself, these thoughts come back.'

'We'll run some tests, just to make sure that you don't have anything serious. In the meantime, I will refer you to a psychologist who you can talk to. It will also be worth your while to take some St. John's Wort. It is a natural supplement that has been shown to help with depression. Since it's a supplement, some brands are better than others, so make sure to get the one I recommend', he told me, writing some notes on a prescription pad. 'Now, Oliver, here is the most important thing', he said, looking me directly in the eye. 'Don't do anything rash, okay? Reach out for help whenever you need it.'

'Okay', I nodded. 'I won't do anything stupid.'

My dad and I drove home. I felt relieved to get my concerns off my chest. In the following days, my appetite began to improve, and I started to sleep better, as well. My mum got me a bottle of St. John's Wort, which seemed to help my mood.

The following week, I made an appointment with the psychologist and went back for a follow up appointment with Dr. Oechsle.

'Good to see you again, Oliver. How are you feeling?' asked the doctor as I walked back into his office.

'I'm feeling much better than I was last week', I replied.

'That's good. You look a lot better today. Have you been having any suicidal thoughts since we last spoke?'

'No', I said, shaking my head. 'Last Thursday was the last time I had those thoughts.'

'That's good to hear. How are you doing at school?'

'I've been feeling better. I'm still a little stressed with the exams, but I'm coping.'

'Excellent. I believe you had an anxiety attack last week, which caused the spiral you went through. I would still like for you to go for a couple of sessions with the psychologist, but it seems that you are doing much better today.'

I attended my first appointment with the psychologist a few weeks later. When I arrived, I did not know what to expect. My psychologist's name was Amanda. She invited me into her office, and after our introductions, she said, 'Now, Oliver, I understand that you have been having issues with your mental health. Do you want to go through with me what you have been feeling?'

'Sure. I've had a lot of concerns that I am about to get seriously ill, brain tumours in particular.'

'Okay, what has caused that concern?' asked Amanda.

'Well, I know a friend of mine who went through that experience, and the thought of it frightened me.' Over the next hour, I explained my concerns in depth, and Amanda helped me to sort through my fears.

I had three more therapy sessions, and eventually I realised that my concerns of having a brain tumour were not based in reality. After that, I chose to stop the psychology sessions and continue to work on my mental health on my own.

After I finished school, I decided to take a year off from studying. During that year, I wanted to spend some time travelling abroad, and I hoped to get into a flight training course.

My anxiety was still high. While I no longer worried about dying of cancer, I now had fears that I wouldn't find the right training course, and that my year would be wasted. My thoughts spun round and round in my mind until one day a few weeks before my birthday, my mum said, 'Oliver, I think I have the perfect birthday gift for you. I spoke to our friend Ben from Qantas, and he has highly recommended the Peninsula Aero Club to train at, so I booked you in for a first flight session.'

'What? Really??' I gasped.

'Yes, you will be flying next Saturday afternoon', said mum.

I trembled with nerves and excitement as I arrived at the Aero Club the following weekend. My family's friend Ben, who is a pilot, was waiting for me by the entrance. 'Oliver! How are you? Good to see you again, mate', said Ben as he reached out to shake my hand.

'Good to see you as well', I said. We made our way over to reception so that I could sign in.

'I'm sure you're looking forward to your first flight session', said Ben.

'I cannot wait', I grinned. As we approached the reception area, another man walked towards me.

'Hi Oliver, I'm Antony, and I will be your instructor for today's flight.'

'Antony, nice to meet you', I replied as I shook his hand. We soon made our way to the tarmac after a quick briefing to begin my first flight session.

'No, you will be in the seat on the left', said Antony as I was about to sit on the right side of the Cessna 152.

'Really? So, I'll be in the captain's seat?' I asked. I could feel my heart beating faster.

'That's right', said Antony. 'I'll be guiding you the whole time, but you are going to be flying the plane.'

I nodded, swallowing hard. It was time to step beyond my comfort zone. As much as my anxiety wanted me to remain on the ground, my desire to fly won out. I climbed into the cockpit and sat down at the controls.

Antony showed me how to start the engine, and then we taxied out to the northern end of the runway. 'Okay, Oliver, grab onto the yoke and gently pull back at 60 knots', said Antony as he applied full throttle. I felt the aircraft lift me powerfully upwards as I pulled a bit too hard on the yoke. A second later, we were climbing into the sky. It was a surreal feeling to finally be at the controls of an aeroplane. It was a dream come true.

> AS I MADE MY WAY BACK TO MY HOUSE AT THE END OF THE SCHOOL DAY, THE DARK CLOUD OVER MY HEAD GREW EVEN LARGER. I FELT THAT I HAD REACHED A BREAKING POINT. THE THOUGHT OF CONTINUING ON BECAME TOO MUCH FOR ME. SOMETHING WITHIN ME URGED ME TO END MY OWN LIFE.

We soared over French Island as part of my introductory flight. Antony was more than impressed with how I handled the plane. 'I have to say, you have a really good feel for the aircraft, especially with the way you're pulling back on the yoke as we're banking', he said.

'Thanks. I've actually been practicing on Microsoft Flight Simulator at home', I replied. 'It's really helped.'

We turned back to Tyabb after flying over French Island for half an hour. After we landed, Ben came over to the aircraft. 'Oliver, how did you go?' asked Ben as I climbed out of the cockpit.

'Apart from a rough take-off, everything went pretty well!' I replied.

'Yeah, I saw your take-off and I thought to myself, oh shit, that had to hurt! Still, you pulled it together', said Ben.

'Yeah, I definitely felt a strong force as we pulled up', I laughed.

'Don't worry about it, Oliver', said Antony. 'You know, you have a really good feel for flying.'

'Thanks, Antony', I said. 'I've got a deep interest in aviation. I've been practicing, and I know I'll get better. I can't wait to fly again.'

I made my way back home after booking another flight lesson for the following weekend. It was clear that the Peninsula Aero Club was going to be my regular spot as I wanted to commit to flying at least once a week.

Ben welcomed me as I arrived for my next session. 'Glad to see you, Oliver! I reckon you're looking forward to your next flight!'

'You betcha!' I grinned. 'I can't wait to learn more.'

'You're getting there! You'll be flying solo in no time', said Ben. 'The hardest part is landing the plane itself. It took me ages to nail that.'

'Yeah, I don't think they'll let me land a plane just yet', I chuckled.

'There is a saying here, Oli—it takes forty shit landings to eventually get one right', laughed Ben. 'At least, that's what it took me.'

'I'll remember that', I smiled.

Two months of weekly training went by. I made a few failed attempts to land the aircraft, but my nerves always got the best of me.

'The trick to executing a landing is to keep your eyes focused on the other end of the runway as you flare out', said Nick, my flight instructor for that day.

As I turned onto final approach and neared closer to the runway, I kept thinking to myself, 'Hold the attitude'. As I touched down, I heard a screech that lasted two seconds. I shook my head. It was another rough landing.

'Not quite there, but you nearly got it', said Nick as I parked the aircraft.

'Oliver, how did you go?' asked Ben as I walked towards the building.

'I don't think I've quite hit the forty shit landings just yet', I laughed. 'I've still got a few more in me before I get it right.'

'You know what, though? You're getting very close', said Nick. 'It takes time to nail the landings, but I don't think you're far off.'

I returned to the Peninsula Aero Club the following weekend for my next lesson with Nick. We took the keys for the Cessna 152 and taxied to the runway to take off. After a few circuits, I prepared to practice my landing.

'Just remember, focus on the end of the runway as you flare out and don't think about the landing too much', said Nick as we turned to finish our first circuit. As I flared out to land, I kept my eyes on the end of the runway, and for the first time, I executed a perfect landing.

'That was brilliant!' said Nick as we took off for another circuit.

'Does this mean that I've surpassed my forty shit landings?' I joked.

Nick chuckled as we continued with our next circuit. I landed again and again after each circuit, and each time, my landings got smoother. Before I knew it, the lesson was over, and we parked the plane.

'You know, Oliver', said Nick, 'I think you're ready to do your first solo. We will be doing that for your next session.'

I left Tyabb feeling high as a kite as I recalled the sensation of my first perfect landing. I was mentally preparing myself for my next hurdle in completing my first solo flight.

The following weekend, I arrived back at the Peninsula Aero Club. Nick greeted me as I walked to reception. 'Oliver! Good to see you, mate. Are you feeling ready for your first solo?'

'Ready as I'll ever be', I said. I felt nervous, but I reminded myself that I knew what I was doing. 'C'mon, Oliver', I told myself. 'Trust your training. You can do this.'

'We'll do a couple of circuits first for safety, and then we'll see where we go from there', said Nick. We both strapped into the Cessna 152 and taxied towards the north of the runway. We took off for one circuit, and again, I was able to execute a perfect landing. 'That's great, Oliver', said Nick. 'We'll do two more circuits, and then we'll have a full stop.'

After we touched down and exited the runway on the third landing, we taxied towards the tarmac. 'Okay, if you can stop for me here, I will get out and you will do your first solo circuit', said Nick. 'Now, when you communicate on radio, say that you are taxiing and departing for your first solo circuit so that the other traffic is aware', Nick added as he disconnected his headset and climbed out of the aircraft. He closed the door and gave me a thumbs up before walking off the tarmac. I did not know how to feel at that point, but I knew that I had to get my first solo done. I wasted no time and contacted Tyabb traffic before I taxied out.

'Traffic Tyabb. Uniform November Delta taxiing to Runway 17 for first solo circuit. Traffic Tyabb', I announced before I taxied out. From this point on, it was all business. I went through the checklists and safety protocols. I was amazed at how easily the aircraft began to move as soon as I released the brake. I realised it was due to the lighter load of having only one person in the cockpit. I arrived at the end of the runway with no inbound traffic in sight, and I knew that it was time for me to commence my take-off.

'Traffic Tyabb. Uniform November Delta lining up and departing Runway 17 for first solo circuit. Traffic Tyabb', I said as I lined up on the runway. It was go time. I focussed my mind, and I put myself into performance mode. Then, I flew.

I felt a rush of exhilaration as I applied full throttle, allowing the aircraft to accelerate down the runway. I pulled back on the yoke and climbed into the sky. As I soared through my circuit, I used my airborne moments to embrace the view of the Mornington Peninsula. I admired the lush greenery that lined the shore, and I marvelled at the glittering water that separated the land from French Island. I was so high up that the ground below looked like a diorama, as if I were a giant walking across a miniature landscape. It was such an adrenaline rush. Every time I turned the aircraft, I felt a jolt of excitement as the wings and engine responded to my commands. It was a powerful feeling to be in control of this machine.

Far too soon, it was time to return to earth. As I commenced my down-wind approach, the conditions were smooth, and I felt no bumps for the duration of my circuit. 'Traffic Tyabb. Uniform November Delta turning final runway 17 for full stop. Traffic Tyabb', I said as I turned to my final approach and prepared for a full-stop landing.

I was determined to pull off another successful landing on my first solo flight. As I began to flare, all I could think about was keeping my eyes on the end of the runway. The aircraft responded to my commands, and I pulled off a textbook landing on my first attempt. I could not stop smiling. I peered over to my right as I taxied back to the stand and saw Nick and Ben waiving. Ben raised his arms up and began clapping as I taxied past. As I shut down the engine, Ben and Nick wasted no time in running towards the plane.

'Oli! Congratulations, mate. That was a brilliant landing', said Ben as he opened my door and reached in to shake my hand.

'Mate. Thanks heaps, I really appreciate it', I replied.

'Oliver, congratulations on completing your first solo!' said Nick as he opened the passenger door.

'Thank you so much', I replied. I felt overwhelmed by their praise. 'I was nervous on how I was going to pull this one off, but I cannot complain', I laughed.

I continued to smile about my achievement for the rest of the day. It allowed me to forget about my depression for a little while. I knew that I was still struggling with my mental health, but for the first time, I believed that I could win this war against my inner demons. Immersing myself in activities that I loved doing helped me turn the tide of the battle.

If you ever feel like life is too much, allow yourself to acknowledge your emotions. If you continue to ignore your struggles, you will only make the situation worse for yourself. Don't be afraid to open up and speak out about how you feel, whether it's to a doctor, your family, or your friends. Being upfront about your battles can be hard, but it's the first step towards a better life. Suicide is never the solution to depression. It ends any chance you have of improving your life, and it causes deep and lasting trauma for your family, your friends, and your community. Trust me when I tell you that recovery from mental illness is possible. Stay on course, and you will get there. There will be turbulence along the way, but you will eventually learn to soar.

ENOUGH IS ENOUGH

During your toughest times, you have two paths that you can choose in life. You can accept things as they are, or you can make changes that will lead to happiness and fulfillment. Taking these actions will necessarily make you feel uncomfortable. Change is by its nature unsettling. However, you will not grow if you stay within your comfort zone. Anxiety and depression often arise when you settle for things, believing that 'it is what it is'. However, there are also times in life where you reach a breaking point. As painful as it may feel, be grateful when you reach this kind of impasse. In these moments, you get to say, 'Enough is enough!' As you read this chapter, I want you to ask yourself, have you ever reached that breaking point? Have you ever stood up, declared 'enough is enough', and then devised a plan of action?

As I continued with my weekly flight training, I was about to embark on a new challenge, which was starting a full-time job. It was exciting for me to move from a part-time position, working less than twenty hours a week in a supermarket, to a full-time, forty-hour-per-week job at a contact centre. Unfortunately, my enthusiasm began to fade three weeks into my new job. Once again, fear began to take over.

'I'm not really sure about this. I'm starting to feel anxious every time I come into work', I confided one day to Erin, a colleague who was always friendly to me.

'You'll be fine, Oliver', said Erin, giving me a sympathetic smile. 'Just don't worry so much. Everything will work out.'

As I logged in that morning, however, my panic began to affect my performance. During the first few calls, I got stuck and didn't know what to say next. I could hear the customers on the other side of the line grow uncomfortable, and one by one, they hung up on me.

'Hey Oliver, is everything alright?' asked Rowena, my manager, as she approached me during my break.

I shrugged my shoulders. 'I just don't feel like I know what I'm doing here in this role. I keep messing up.'

'You only just started here, so it's perfectly normal to make mistakes', smiled Rowena, trying to reassure me. 'If we notice errors in your work, we will just let you know what went wrong and explain what you need to do next time. Don't worry, Oliver. We have a protocol for this.'

'Okay. Yeah, I just need to calm down', I nodded as I forced myself to take a deep breath.

Rowena reached out and patted my shoulder. 'Don't stress. You're going to be fine.'

I sighed as Rowena turned and walked back to her desk. It was kind of her to try and comfort me, but instead of reassurance, I felt even more anxiety. What if she thought that I was a burden? I didn't see anyone else at work confessing to her about their fear of making mistakes. I tried hard to calm myself, but despite my efforts, I continued to feel my heart beating through my chest.

Two years passed. I stayed in my full-time role at the company, despite my constant anxiety that I would be fired. Slowly, the dark cloud that had hung over me in high school began to return. I felt depressed, and I couldn't see any light in my life.

'Hey Oliver, how are you doing, mate?' asked Andy, my work colleague, as we walked to the breakout room for tea.

I could hear a note of concern in his voice. 'I'm okay', I replied, trying to sound cheerful, though I don't think I was fooling anyone.

'You sure?' Andy pressed.

'I don't know. I haven't really been myself lately. I've just been feeling really down. It's like I can't even imagine myself being happy', I confessed, letting out a long sigh.

Andy patted me on the back. 'I'm sorry, Oliver. That sounds really difficult. I'm sure it'll pass eventually.'

'I hope it does', I nodded. 'It's getting to a point where I'm struggling to get out of bed.'

Andy paused for a moment, then he asked me, 'Have you ever thought of talking to someone about it? Like a therapist?'

I nodded my head distractedly, mumbling, 'Yeah, I'll have to look into that.' That conversation with Andy planted a seed in my mind. Later that week, I called a psychologist to schedule an appointment.

I started calling out sick from work on a regular basis, citing personal reasons for my absences. Soon, management became concerned. My manager, Danielle, called me into her office one morning.

'Hey Oliver, I have notice you've been taking a lot of sick days lately. Is everything okay?'

I looked at my hands and sighed. 'I haven't been well lately, to be honest.'

Danielle leaned forward in her chair, looking concerned. 'Do you want to tell me what is going on?'

'I've just been having a lot of issues with my anxiety lately. It's affecting my day-to-day life.' I passed my hand across my brow, noticing that my forehead was clammy.

'I'm really sorry to hear that, Oliver', said Danielle, giving me a compassionate look. 'Is there anything we can do to support you?'

I took a deep breath. 'I think I'll need certain days off', I said. 'Though some of these can be half days. I've reached out to a specialist to help me with my anxiety. I'm meeting with her regularly.'

'Okay, we can accommodate that', nodded Danielle. 'You'll need to let us know which days you'll be taking off in advance.'

'Thank you. I really appreciate this. I like it here a lot, and I want to keep working here. I just need to get my anxiety under control.'

I wanted to feel relieved, but getting called into the manager's office only caused my anxiety to spike. I was more terrified than ever of being laid off.

Time wore on, and I noticed that my mum had started taking time off work. I was concerned because she rarely took sick days. I asked her if anything was wrong, and what she told me caused my anxiety to climb even higher. 'I've been having some stomach troubles. But please, don't worry, Oliver.' A few months passed, and mum's pain began to get worse. I would often see her doubled over, clutching her stomach. One day, she told me, 'Oliver, I don't want you to worry, but I'm going to see a doctor tomorrow. He's going to find out what's wrong. It will all be okay, I promise.' A week later, she was referred to an oncologist, and a few days after that, she sat me down after dinner. She looked scared, but she was trying to put on a brave face. 'Oliver, I just found out that I'm going in for surgery tomorrow. They found a growth in my abdomen.' Her voice wobbled. I felt like I had just been punched in the gut. I didn't know what to say or do. I was terrified.

The following evening, mum was admitted to Cabrini Hospital for her surgery. My dad and I sat by the phone as the night wore on, anxiously awaiting a call from the doctor. Finally, the phone rang. My father answered. He was on the call for about five minutes. Finally, he hung up and turned to face me. He looked shaken. 'Oliver, that was the surgeon. They have found cancer in her ovaries. She'll spend a few days in hospital, and then she'll need to start chemotherapy. But it's not all bad news. The doctor said that her prognosis is good. Please, Oliver, don't worry. She's going to beat this.'

My heart sank. I felt my mind go numb. It was as if I were frozen in place. I did not know what to do. How was I going to handle my mother battling cancer? What would I do if she never recovered? I was terrified that she was going to die. My stomach churned. It felt like I had swallowed a live coal.

From that moment, my life began spiralling out of control. I fell deeper into my depression. I stopped caring about my mindset and my body, not that I had cared much before. I quit my therapy sessions. I relied mainly on takeaway and junk food, which started to take a serious toll on my health. I was on a downhill slope to nowhere good.

My mum was disturbed. Even though she was sick from chemotherapy, she noticed my distress. 'Oliver, I'm worried about you. I want you to eat dinner with us more often so that you're not eating takeaway all the time.' My dad also noticed the changes. 'Oliver, you look like you've started putting on weight. I'm concerned about your health.' I told them both that I would try my best to change my habits, but I didn't know how.

I fell into a pattern of eating junk food and takeaway. It was difficult for me to change my behaviour, even after my mum finished her chemotherapy and was declared cancer-free. Over the next few years, my eating and drinking habits got progressively worse. As I continued to gain weight, my clothing budget increased, as well. Every six months or so, I would have to buy a new wardrobe to accommodate my increasing size. Each time I looked in the mirror, I felt more and more ashamed of the person I saw looking back at me. These feelings of shame eroded my self-esteem, and my depression became even worse. I was caught in a vicious cycle.

Soon, I began to shut myself off from the world. I felt uncomfortable socializing with large groups, let alone engaging in personal conversations. I still received invitations to social events, but I declined almost every one at the last minute because 'I had other plans'. On nights when I was required to attend social functions for work, I would leave within an hour of arriving. I felt like a stranger in my own skin.

In 2014, I reached a breaking point. I realised that if I continued on this path in life, I would wind up in an early grave. I was miserable and sick. I said to myself, 'Enough is enough. I need to find help.' I reached out to a life coach to at least start the process of rebuilding my confidence.

My coach's name was Tim. He was a charismatic man with a warm smile. In our first session, we met at a café in Chadstone. After we ordered our tea, Tim turned to me and asked, 'So, Oliver, tell me—what are the key areas that you wish to work on in your life?'

'I-I want to rebuild my self-esteem', I stammered, looking down at my hands. 'I have completely lost confidence in myself. I can't seem to start a conversation without feeling nervous.'

Tim nodded, seeming to scrutinise my downturned face. 'Okay. Now, when you say that you can't seem to start a conversation with someone, is it anyone in particular?'

I shook my head. 'Pretty much anyone, but mainly women, to be honest. I want to have a happy relationship, but I struggle to even meet with people. How in the world am I supposed to go on a date with a woman if I can't even talk to her?'

'Okay', said Tim, nodding his head thoughtfully. 'What is it that you are worried about when you talk to a woman?'

I squirmed in my chair. 'I'm afraid that she will think that I am a loser, and that she won't want me around', I said, glancing up at Tim. He gave me a compassionate smile.

'Thank you, Oliver', he said. 'I really appreciate you being open and honest about this. But let me ask you this. When you approach a woman, how do you know that she is thinking those things?'

I sat in silence, my mind spinning. After what felt like several minutes, Tim said, 'I can see that you are struggling to find the answer to that question. The reality is that you can't read someone's mind to determine what they are thinking. In fact, no one can.'

I considered this for a moment. 'I guess that's true', I muttered.

Tim continued. 'I can completely understand how you are feeling, having a lack of confidence. Believe it or not, I was the least confident person that you could imagine when I was younger. It took me a lot of work and a lot of help to get to where I am today. I am going to use all the tools that I learned to help you build your confidence.'

Over the next several sessions, Tim introduced me to Neuro-Linguistic Programming exercises to progressively build up my self-esteem. One day, he announced, 'Okay, Oliver, we are going to begin taking the next steps. We are going to go out there and start talking to people.'

'Are we doing this right now?' I asked, feeling a knot form in the pit of my stomach.

'We sure are', grinned Tim. 'Let's head over to Melbourne Central.'

My heart began to pound. This was everything I was afraid of. I did not feel ready to have conversations with strangers. By the time we arrived in Melbourne Central, my heart was racing, and my forehead was covered with sweat. Tim gave me a pat on the back. 'I want you to go out there and start a conversation with any girl you see.'

I felt like I wanted to crawl under a rock and never emerge again, but I mustered up enough courage to say, 'Okay, I'll give it a try.

We walked around Melbourne Central for fifteen or twenty minutes.'

Eventually, I tried walking up to a woman, but I panicked as I approached her, and she hurried past me.

"

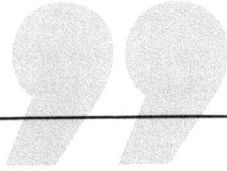

IN THE VICIOUS CYCLE OF
ANXIETY AND DEPRESSION,
THE HIGHEST OF HIGHS ARE
OFTEN FOLLOWED BY THE
LOWEST OF LOWS. AFTER A
FEW DAYS, I WAS BACK TO
FEELING UNFULFILLED AND
HOPELESS.

Tim walked over and asked, 'Hey, Oliver, is everything alright? We've been here for a while now, and you haven't said a word to anyone.'

'I'm really struggling, to be honest', I told him, wiping my forehead on my sleeve. 'I don't know what to say when I approach people. I kind of feel like I might be sick.'

'Okay, let's make this easier', suggested Tim. 'Why don't you start by asking a simple question, like, "Where is the Optus store?" How does that feel?'

'Okay, that might be easier for me', I nodded.

I took Tim's suggestion and walked around asking random pedestrians for the location of the Optus store. Most of the people simply pointed and went on their way. A few people, however, asked me some questions about what I needed. This flustered me again. I got nervous and didn't know what to do. I think I stammered something and walked away.

Tim could tell that I was close to my breaking point. He walked up to me and said, 'Hey, Oliver, you seem a little anxious.'

'Yeah, I-I don't feel comfortable doing this at all', I stammered, wiping my sweaty brow.

'That's good', grinned Tim. 'We want to get you out of your comfort zone. That is where personal growth happens. The further away from your comfort zone you go, the better your life becomes. We are going to be doing more of this over the next couple of weeks. After that, we are going to sign you up for speed dating.'

I felt sick to my stomach, but I trusted Tim. After all, he had been through this process himself. If he could do it, so could I.

We returned to Melbourne Central two weeks later and continued our exercise in engaging in conversation. 'Same deal as last time', said Tim as we scanned the crowd. 'This will help improve your confidence.'

I walked toward the busy sidewalk and began speaking to strangers. 'Hi, do you know where the Optus store is?'

I happened to say this to a woman walking by. She stopped and turned to face me. 'Yes, I think it's just down the escalators near the big clock.'

I don't know what courage came over me, but I replied, 'Thanks! And I have to say that I love your accent! Are you by any chance from the US?'

'Oh, thank you', she laughed. 'No, I'm actually from Ireland.'

I think I blushed, though my face was already red from nerves. 'Oh, sorry. For some reason, I thought your accent was American.'

'Yes, I get that a lot', she smiled. 'Nice to meet you.' She turned and continued walking down the street.

Tim came over to me, smiling broadly. 'Oliver, I have to say that you did an awesome job talking to that girl. You had a genuine back-and-forth conversation with her. I can see your confidence growing. This is a big step forward.'

'Yeah, I don't know what just happened', I smiled, 'but I am happy with the way it went.'

Tim clapped me on the shoulder. 'You should be! When I saw you, I was like, oh, where did THAT Oliver come from?'

Tim and I left Melbourne Central after twenty minutes, calling it a day. As we walked back toward the tram, he said, 'I believe that you are ready to take the next step. For our next session, we will move onto speed dating. It will be a challenge, but I know for sure that it will build your confidence.'

The next week, Tim and I met up at the speed dating venue in the city. Tim clapped me on the shoulder, reassuring me, 'You've got this. Just remember to maintain eye contact. When you talk, all you have to do is respond, elaborate, and ask.'

I nodded, trying to swallow. My mouth was so dry, it felt like I was swallowing a desert. 'Okay. Eye contact, right. I'm pretty nervous, but I'm ready to take this step.'

We walked into the venue, and I signed in. The night went by in a blur. I talked to about twelve women, and each 'date' lasted sixty seconds. The moderator rang a bell after each minute was up so we would know to start talking to the next person. I didn't have time to think or be nervous. I know I was awkward, but no one seemed to notice. All the women I spoke to were probably so preoccupied with managing their own anxiety that they didn't care about mine. I even had a few short conversations with some of the women during the coffee break.

Tim caught up with me after the event. 'How did it go tonight?' he asked.

'I actually had a lot of fun', I grinned.

Tim patted my shoulder. 'That's awesome, Oliver. I'll be taking you to a few more of these events. They will help you overcome your social anxiety.'

'Okay', I nodded, taking a deep breath. 'That's cool. I'm actually kind of looking forward to the next one.'

Unfortunately, in the journey of life, there will always be setbacks. After attending three more speed dating events, I found myself backing away from social occasions and returning to my unhealthy habits. I think I was moving a bit too quickly in my quest to discover my confidence. A little too much 'fake it' and not enough 'make it'. Over the next two years, I continued to gain more weight. Eventually, I did not even recognize myself. I fell into a deep pit with a dark cloud hanging over me.

Just when I thought I was lost forever in depression and anxiety, friendship brought me back from the brink. I met my friend Sheetal through a social event. She and I kept in touch, and a few months later, she invited me to an event that her family was hosting. It was a fundraiser for the Australian Integrated Fijian Association of Victoria. By now, I worked in superannuation, which was a stressful position in my company, and I looked forward to a break from work. When I arrived, Sheetal introduced me to her uncle Rohit and her aunt Shalini. They were kind and inquisitive, and they seemed to take a genuine interest in me. I basked in their attention. I sat through the show, appreciating the Indian Fijian culture. I was impressed by the effort that AIFAV put in to make sure that the show was a success.

The next day, I was inspired to record a live video, promoting the upcoming shows that AIFAV was sponsoring. I don't quite know what gave me the courage to do it. Perhaps it was the gratitude that I felt toward Sheetal's family for welcoming me into their group. My voice shook as I looked at the camera. I gasped and stammered, trying for the life of me not to be overcome with anxiety. As I spoke, I decided to share my story. I told the viewers that I had been diagnosed with Severe Language Disorder as a child, and that even as an adult, communication was difficult for me. As terrifying as it was to talk to this unseen audience, I knew that this fear was something that I needed to overcome. As I spoke, I remembered Tim's words. I told the viewers that I needed to step outside of my comfort zone in order to grow.

> 'ENOUGH IS ENOUGH!' I TOLD MYSELF. I KNEW I NEEDED TO CHANGE, BUT ON THAT DAY, I FINALLY ACCEPTED THAT THE ONLY PERSON CAPABLE OF MAKING THAT CHANGE WAS ME.

Sheetal's aunt Shalini reached out to me over Facebook later that day. She wrote, 'Dear Oliver, you have touched our hearts with your speech. Thank you for sharing your story.'

From then on, I developed a close friendship with Sheetal, Rohit, and Shalini. They became some of my dearest friends. Sheetal was one of the first people that I told of my bucket list plan for my thirtieth birthday. I had always loved airplanes. It didn't matter whether I was flying them or flying in them, I exalted in the freedom of the open sky. Still, there was one thing that I had never done before. I had never jumped out of a plane. This year, I was going to treat myself to a trip to California to go skydiving. It would be the ultimate adventure.

I booked my flight to Los Angeles. I was going to skydive in nearby Perris, California, which was two hours east of LA by car. Sheetal had scheduled a trip to Santa Monica at around the same time, so we planned to meet up there two days after I landed. Before I knew it, the day arrived for me to board my flight to LAX. I strategically didn't sleep the night before so I could get some rest on the flight. I was excited to fly on the impressive, 250-seat United Boeing 787-9 Dreamliner. It is a majestic airplane. The wonder of flight brought me back to my childhood, when I first experienced the freedom of soaring unfettered through the sky. As I boarded the plane and waited for the cabin doors to close, I realised that no one else was sitting in my row. I smiled to myself. My luck and strategy had paid off. I would be able to stretch out and get comfortable. I managed to get six hours of decent sleep on the flight and woke in LA without much jetlag.

I rented a car and drove up to Santa Monica. I was excited to see Sheetal. A couple days later, we met up for lunch. Afterwards, we walked along the pier, chatting about my birthday and my upcoming skydive.

'Are you nervous?' asked Sheetal.

I thought for a moment. 'Yeah, a little', I confessed. 'Not so much about jumping, actually. I guess I'm anxious that I'm about to cross off a major item from my bucket list. It feels like a reminder that I haven't lived the life that

I wanted to. I'm about to turn thirty, and I'm honestly wondering if all the decisions I've made are wrong.'

'I know you'll figure this out, Oliver', said Sheetal as she reached out to touch my arm, her eyes brimming with compassion. 'You've been through a lot in your life. But you've got friends here to help you through this. Please, let us in. Let us help you.'

We walked in silence for a while. I could tell that Sheetal was concerned about me, which made me nervous. I didn't want her to decide that I was too much for her to handle. I felt like a burden. I began spiralling into another bout of depression. I told myself to pull it together. Tomorrow was a big day. I was going to jump into the sky. It would be my chance to let go of old fears and take the first steps into a new life. That's what I hoped for, anyway.

The next morning, I got into my rental car and drove southeast. After two hours on the road, I arrived at a very wet Perris, which had been drenched by a heavy rainstorm that morning. I pulled into the parking lot of the tiny Perris Valley Airport and quickly located the office of Skydive Perris, the company that would be taking me into the sky that day. The clerk informed me that there would be a delay due to the weather. 'No problem', I replied. There was no way I was backing out now. After an hour's wait, the clerk called me over to watch an instructional video about skydiving and sign a liability waiver. I agreed not to hold them at fault if I experienced injury or death. The reality of what I was about to do came into stark focus. The clerk interrupted my thoughts before I could chicken out.

'What's the occasion for making the jump?' he asked.

'I'm doing this to celebrate my thirtieth birthday', I replied as I handed him the sheet of paper that had suddenly made me aware of my mortality.

'Oh, happy birthday! We'll give you $40 off', smiled the clerk.

My jaw dropped. 'Oh wow! Thank you so much!' This seemed like a good omen.

Another hour went by, and I was called into the hangar to suit up for the jump. A man in skydiving gear approached me.

'Oliver?' he yelled over the loud roar of airplane engines.

'Yes, that's me!' I shouted.

'I'm Craig', smiled the man. 'I'll be your skydiving instructor. Nice to meet you.'

We shook hands, and Craig helped me get into my gear. The nerves really started to kick in as Craig and I boarded the twin prop aircraft and strapped our harnesses together. There were several other people making the jump today. Craig and I sat down near the exit, and soon we were rolling down the runway. I felt increasingly anxious as we took to the sky, climbing higher and higher into the wild blue yonder. I was concerned that my heart might pound through my chest. A lump formed in my throat, making it difficult to swallow. A few minutes later, we reached our final altitude of 12,500 feet. One of the instructors threw the door open. Craig and I were closest to the exit, so we were the first to jump. Just my luck, I thought. I leaned over the edge, breathing heavily as I looked down at the earth, which now resembled a distant green and brown patchwork quilt.

Craig leaned us forward, then back, and then forward again. The momentum was enough to propel us out of the plane. We made the leap. As we began to freefall, I looked up, and for a moment it seemed like the plane above us was shooting straight into the sky. I knew that this was merely an optical illusion. We were actually plummeting downward at a breathtaking rate. After a minute or so, Craig opened the parachute, and we began to level out. I couldn't help but smile. That leap I took was the leap of freedom. For a moment, I felt liberated from the past twenty-nine years. Deep down, I knew I was capable of doing anything.

'How are you feeling?' Craig yelled into my ear as we glided downward toward the airfield.

'Well, no piss, no shit, and no vomit, so I'm doing great!' I yelled back, grinning ear to ear. As we landed back on the field, I knew that I had achieved a huge milestone.

I felt incredibly proud of myself for what I had accomplished that day. In the evening, I called my family and friends back in Australia to describe the experience. I could barely contain the excitement that I was feeling. The company emailed me a video of the jump, which I watched over and over as I sat in my hotel room, reliving the magic of the day.

Sadly, the happiness and excitement did not last long. In the vicious cycle of anxiety and depression, the highest of highs are often followed by the lowest of lows. After a few days, I was back to feeling unfulfilled and hopeless. I didn't see the point of continuing on this way, and I considered suicide. With the benefit of hindsight, I can see that I may have just been exhausted from the stress of travel. Depression and anxiety often trick us into believing that the normal experience of stress is unmanageable and something that we can never overcome.

As I concluded my trip and flew back to Melbourne, I knew that I had to make a major change in my life. I was stuck in a state of perpetual unhappiness. I felt ashamed of myself because of my weight. When I returned to the office later that week, my colleague Kris asked me if I wanted to take part in a workplace challenge. I didn't know what it was for, but I reckoned why not. I didn't have anything else going for me, did I? Kris forwarded me an email from the organiser. The title read, 'Biggest Loser Competition'. As I read the contents of the email, I saw it was an invitation to an office weight loss competition. I shook my head. I told myself that even if I tried my hardest to lose weight, I would fail. After all, I had never succeeded before.

I was about to hit delete, but something within me stopped my hand. Instead, I typed, 'I'm in.' Then I hit send.

'Enough is enough!' I told myself. I knew I needed to change, but on that day, I finally accepted that the only person capable of making that change was me.

There are occasions in life where you are given an opportunity to be a part of something that will alter the course of your future. If you receive an invitation to an event, a group, or a challenge, don't hide behind a wall of fear and shame. Instead, say yes. It may change your life. If you find that it is not for you, there is no shame in walking away, but either way, it will help you grow. If you have an item on your bucket list that you have always wanted to do, find a way to make it happen. Let me put it this way, at the end of your life, do you really want to say, 'Why didn't I go for it?' Wouldn't you rather say, 'I am so glad I did it!' Have a think about it. Which way do you want to go? The choice is entirely up to you.

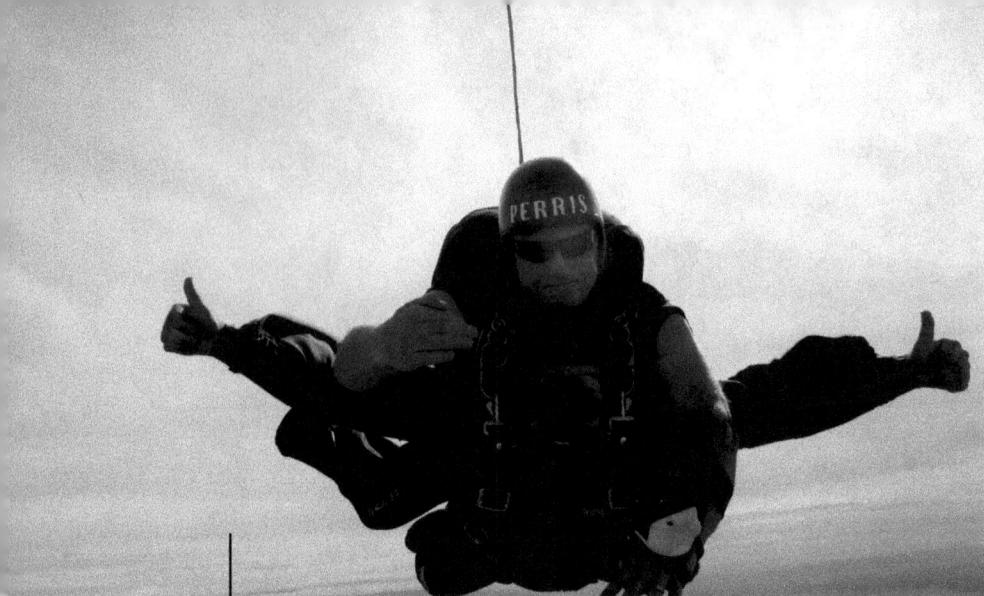

Skydiving — This was when I was freefalling from 12,500ft over Perris, California during my first skydive. Photographer — Unknown

Gym training — During my one-on-one session with my personal trainer, William. We were focusing on building shoulder strength in the photo. Photographer — Mark Banta

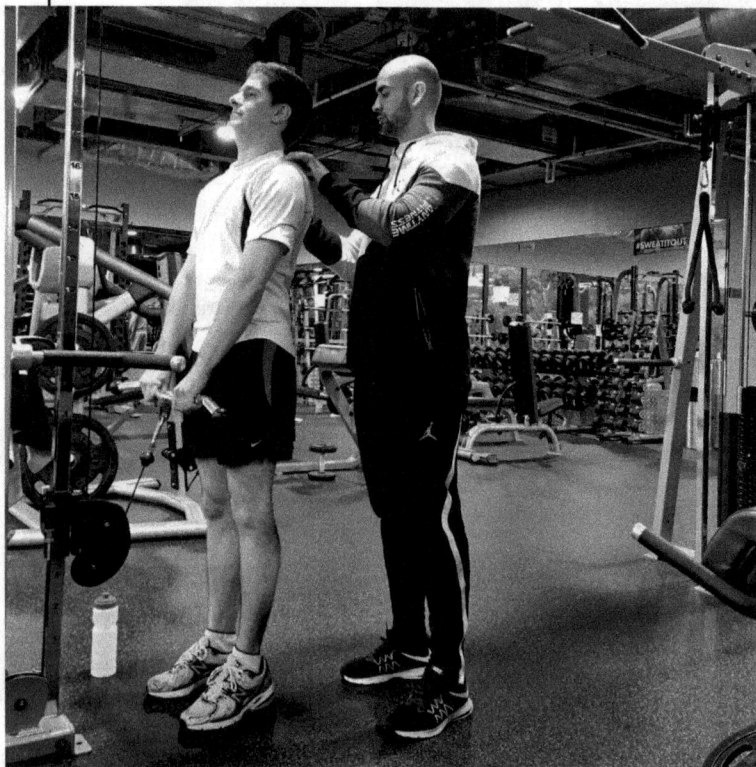

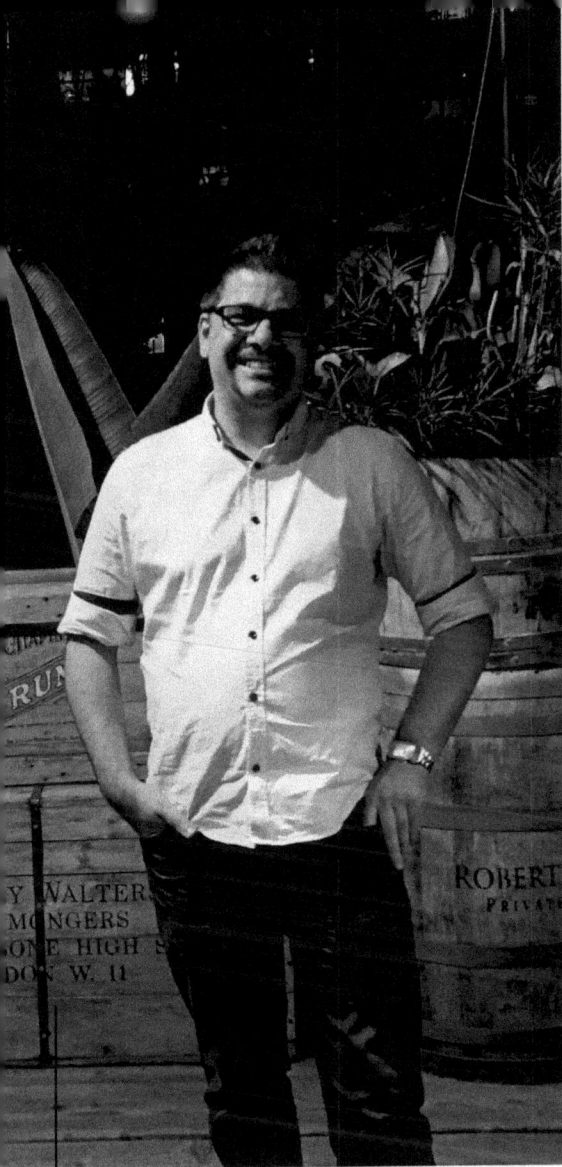

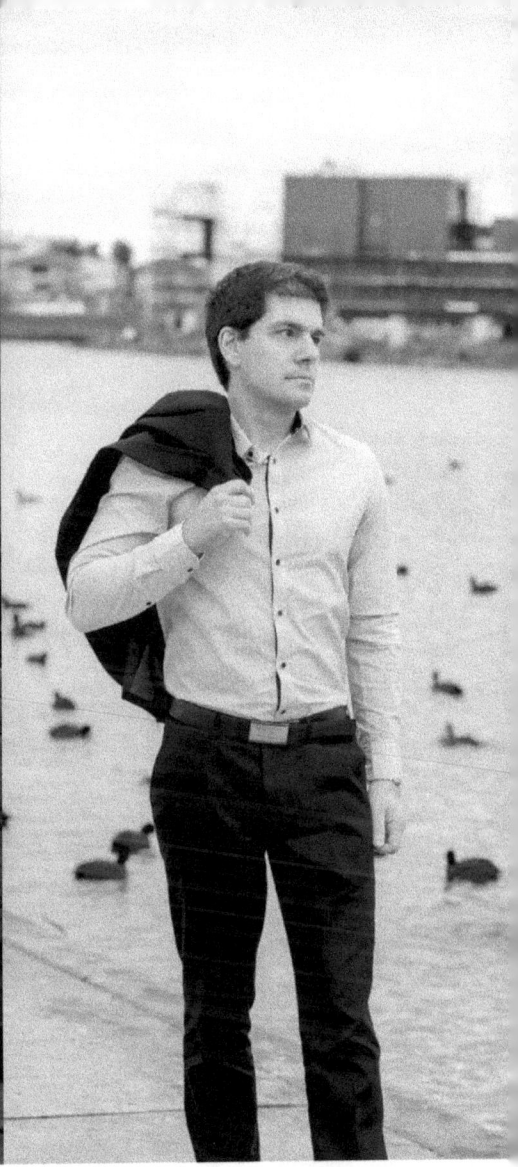

Before and after — Photo on the left was during my visit to California, shortly before I decided to make the lifestyle change. Photo on the right was during my photoshoot in Brimbank Park. The weight loss between the two photos was 22kg. Photographer (left photo) — Sheetal Ashika Singh. Photographer (right photo) — Safia Sahib

CHAPTER

04

THE START OF A NEW BEGINNING

When we reach a moment of breakthrough and decide to turn our life around, it's normal to ask questions like, 'How am I going to get started?' and 'How long will I be able to maintain my momentum?' A question that I often asked myself was, 'Will this new lifestyle work for me in the long run?' In the past, whenever I had made a change, it had never taken me long to return to my old habits. I would give up far too soon and start bingeing on food and drink, which would lead me right back to the hole that I had just crawled out of. There is a wise old saying that states, 'Wherever you go, there you are'. What this means is that you will keep repeating the same patterns until you make the conscious decision to change your behaviour. I desperately wanted to be happy and healthy, but I had always sought to alter my outside circumstances, hoping that this time, things would go my way. The one thing I hadn't yet tried to change was my mindset. This time, I knew that I had to step up to the challenge. No one else was going to come and save me. It was my responsibility alone to transform my life.

After I accepted the invitation to participate in the Biggest Loser challenge, I struggled to picture the end goal of what I wanted to achieve. I imagined myself as a slim, healthy man, but I didn't know how I would get there. That's when I realised that appearance wasn't the best metric to use. Instead, I decided to use health to measure my success. I wanted to look at myself in the mirror and say to myself, 'Oliver, I'm proud of you for making healthy choices'. I started taking small steps towards this goal. Instead of ordering deep-fried, takeaway meals, I would eat grilled chicken and salad. Instead of gulping down a soft drink, I would have a glass of water. After only a few weeks, I started to feel noticeably healthier.

'Are you going to look around for a gym that you want to join?' asked my colleague Kris one afternoon.

'I think I might join the gym here in Collins Square', I replied.

'Do you mean Anytime Fitness?' asked Kris.

'Yes, that's the place. I had a look at their reviews, and I liked what people had to say.'

'That's cool', said Kris. 'I'm planning on joining the one near where I live. It has enough for me in terms of equipment and classes.'

'I'm glad you have a place in mind', I said. 'I think I'll need some structure, so I might look into getting a personal trainer to help me.'

These were small steps, but I knew it was a start. I reckoned that I would be intimidated to tour the gym alone, so I made an appointment to see the gym manager. As soon as I secured a time online to visit Anytime Fitness, I felt a wave of excitement wash over me. I sensed that I was on the cusp of a profound transformation. As soon as I finished work that afternoon, I headed down to the gym, which was just a few doors over in the same square.

As I walked through the glass door, I made eye contact with a man inside who was managing the front desk.

'Hello, how are you doing today?' asked the man as I approached the reception area.

'I'm very well, thank you', I replied. 'My name is Oliver. I made an appointment to see the gym today.'

'Oh, yes, Oliver. Such a pleasure to meet you. I'm Phil. I'm the club owner and manager. Let me show you around the facility.'

Phil shook my hand and led me around the gym, describing the amenities that it had to offer. After a brief tour, I knew that I wanted to get started.

'Just letting you know, there is a seven-day free trial', Said Phil. 'If you are happy with everything, we would love for you to be a member.'

'That sounds really good to me', I replied. 'I'm happy to sign the paperwork and start training tomorrow.'

'Fantastic! Let's get you signed up', said Phil. 'I'm looking forward to seeing your transformation here!'

The next day, I brought my gym clothing with me to my job so that I could head straight to Anytime Fitness after work. As soon as my shift ended, I went down to the gym, changed into my gear, and looked around the space. I didn't know what I should start with, so I decided to begin by jogging on the treadmill. I aimed for a ten-minute run. It was much harder than I had anticipated. I had to take breaks every thirty seconds or so. I would turn the speed down, walk for a few seconds, and then speed back up to a jog. Although I struggled, I kept pushing through. At the end of the ten minutes, I felt accomplished for having reached this first fitness goal.

After my warmup on the treadmill, I decided to work on my upper body, mainly my biceps. I spent an hour lifting weights before heading to the locker room. I changed back into my work attire and got ready to return home. On my way out, I stopped by the manager's office. Phil sat at the desk, completing some paperwork. I knocked on the open doorframe.

'How did your first training go?' asked Phil as he looked up from his computer.

'It went very well. Definitely worked hard today', I replied. 'I can't wait to get started on my journey.'

'Good on you!' said Phil. 'Just so you know, as part of your sign-up package, you have a complimentary one-on-one session with a personal trainer, if you're interested in going down that path.'

'That sounds great', I replied. 'I don't really know what I'm doing yet.'

'You will be amazed at how beneficial it will be to have a personal trainer to help you', said Phil. 'I will arrange for you to work with Mark. He's one of our best!'

The following day, I was scheduled for my complimentary one-on-one session. I made my way to Anytime Fitness with a mixture of anticipation and nerves. I was ready for fitness coaching, but at the same time, I was unsure of what I was about to endure. Mark, my trainer, met me at the gym and brought me to the personal trainers' office in the back of the facility.

'Good to meet you, Oliver', said Mark. 'Before we get into our session, I want to go through your fitness goals.'

'Well, there are a few things', I replied. 'I want to build strength and increase my muscle tone. I'm also looking to lose weight.'

'Those are good objectives. Just so that I know how best to help you, could you tell me about your weight loss goals?' asked Mark.

'Well, I'm participating in a weight loss competition that a friend of mine organised at work. My aim is to lose 20kg.'

'Okay', said Mark. 'My advice for you is to not weigh yourself too frequently. I'm going to recommend that you go by how your clothes fit. It's best not to get too fixated on the numbers on the scale.'

'That might be difficult', I said. 'I do need to weigh myself on a weekly basis to send in the weight loss results.'

'Okay, well how about we weigh you here at the gym once a week?'

'That would work, so long as I can report the numbers to the organiser.'

'What sort of competition is this, if you don't mind my asking?'

'It's a Biggest Loser competition that I decided to join. I haven't done anything like this before, but I figured that I might as well give it a go. I think it will give me good motivation to get in shape.'

'Okay, well, I know that personal coaching will be able to help you stay motivated during the process. It will also help you achieve your goals safely. We want to make sure that your weekly and monthly weight loss objectives are reasonable.'

After Mark talked with me about my goals, he took me onto the gym floor to begin our first circuit. I didn't know what kind of exercises Mark was going to have me do, but I told myself that no matter what, I was going to get through my first session.

'Okay, Oliver', said Mark. 'We are going to train in the circuit area and do four different exercises. We are going to do push-ups, squats, plank, and burpees. We'll do each exercise for thirty seconds, and we'll have a thirty-second break in between rounds.' Mark got down on the floor and demonstrated one round of the exercise circuit.

THERE IS A WISE OLD SAYING THAT STATES, 'WHEREVER YOU GO, THERE YOU ARE'. WHAT THIS MEANS IS THAT YOU WILL KEEP REPEATING THE SAME PATTERNS UNTIL YOU MAKE THE CONSCIOUS DECISION TO CHANGE YOUR BEHAVIOUR.

I felt the colour drain from my face. 'That doesn't look easy, but I will give it a shot', I replied. I was nervous but still excited to try.

'You will be fine. I'll be here to guide you', said Mark.

I knew that it was going to be a challenging first session, but I was determined to persevere.

'Okay, Oliver. Are you ready?' asked Mark as he set up the timer.

'I'm good to go', I nodded, as I lowered my body into push-up position.

'Your thirty seconds starts...now!' said Mark as I shakily lowered myself to the floor as far as I could go. 'Come on, Oliver! Use those arms!' encouraged Mark as I strained to push myself away from the ground. 'Give it all you got. You got this!'

As I completed my first set of push-ups, I struggled to catch my breath. Gasping for air, I reached for my towel to wipe my face and neck, which were starting to drip with sweat.

'Alright! Get ready for your first set of squats!' said Mark as he reset the timer.

'Okay', I nodded. 'I'm ready. No excuses.'

'That's the attitude I want to see, Oliver', said Mark. 'Just get through this, and you'll be fine. Ready? And go!'

I got through my first few squats comfortably before I started feeling a burning sensation in my quads. My legs began to tremble, and I worried that my knees might give out.

'Come on Oliver! Don't slow down now!' said Mark as I pushed through the pain with the last few seconds remaining. 'And stop. Well done.'

'Wow, this is not easy', I panted.

'This first circuit will be hard, but you'll get through it, I promise you. Next up is plank.'

I nodded and got down on all fours as Mark showed me the correct planking posture.

'Okay, ready? Your thirty seconds of planking starts...now!' Mark started the timer, and I got into plank position. 'I want to see your hips higher', said Mark. The burning sensation I felt in my core began to intensify as I struggled to keep from collapsing.

'And time! How did that feel?' asked Mark as I gasped for air.

'I'm starting to hurt a little bit everywhere', I replied. I tried to chuckle, but it came out as a cough.

'Good! You will have fun with burpees', said Mark as he gave me a cheeky smile.

'I don't know if I like your idea of fun', I laughed as Mark demonstrated a few burpees.

'You'll thank me when you win your work competition. You've got this! Thirty seconds of burpees starts...now!' said Mark.

I started out at a good pace, but I began to slow down halfway through. I had never done burpees before, and I had no idea how challenging it could be to combine push-ups with jumps. I felt my triceps and shoulders burning as I pushed myself up and leapt towards the ceiling, reaching my arms overhead as I jumped.

'Come on! You got this Oliver!' shouted Mark as I got down to the last few seconds. 'And stop! Good job, buddy', said Mark as he reached out his hand to shake mine.

'Now, we are going to do it all over again', said Mark. I must have looked pale because Mark added, 'Don't worry, we're going to take a couple of minutes between sets. Take some deep breaths and have a drink of water.'

I wiped my brow and gulped down nearly half my water bottle. Then I assumed my position, ready to do my next set of push-ups. 'Okay, I'm ready! Let's do this!'

'That's the attitude! Okay, thirty seconds of push-ups. And go!'

> I COMPLETED TWO MORE ROUNDS OF THE EXERCISE CIRCUIT. I WORKED MYSELF TO NEAR EXHAUSTION, BUT I FELT A HUGE SENSE OF ACCOMPLISHMENT AS SOON AS I FINISHED MY FINAL SET. EVEN THOUGH I STRUGGLED THROUGH THE LAST CIRCUIT, I KEPT MY PROMISE TO MYSELF THAT I WOULD NOT GIVE UP. 'ENOUGH IS ENOUGH', I THOUGHT TO MYSELF. 'NO MORE EXCUSES.'

I completed two more rounds of the exercise circuit. I worked myself to near exhaustion, but I felt a huge sense of accomplishment as soon as I finished my final set. Even though I struggled through the last circuit, I kept my promise to myself that I would not give up. 'Enough is enough', I thought to myself. 'No more excuses.'

As I wiped my face with my towel, Mark patted me on the back. 'Congratulations, Oliver! You did great in this first session.'

'Thanks, Mark', I replied whilst catching my breath. 'It was not easy, but I got the job done.'

'Good work', said Mark. 'Now, I would like you to do the same circuit you just learned at least three times a week.'

'Yep, will do', I nodded.

Christmastime was just around the corner. I knew that in addition to my regular workouts at the gym, I needed to make some major changes to the way I ate if I wanted to compete in my workplace challenge. I needed to fight the temptation to eat red meat, and I needed to add more fruits and vegetables to my diet. After having a dinner one night that consisted of fish and veggies, I realized that by chance I'd just had a meat free day. I remembered a friend of mine who followed a pescatarian diet. Instead of meat and poultry, he ate fish. I decided that I would try this path. I knew it would help with my weight-loss journey, and I reckoned it would also be satisfying. If I got to eat a delicious salmon fillet for dinner each night, I would be less tempted to sneak in a cheat meal.

Soon, it was New Year's Day, 2018. I knew that this was my year to make a change for the better. A few days into January, I walked into Anytime Fitness and got ready to practice the routine that Mark had taught me. As I made my way through the gym, I decided to pop in to say hi to Phil in the manager's office.

'Hey, Phil', I said as I knocked on his open door.

'Hey matey, how are you? You're looking great! I can see a difference already, and it's only been a few weeks since you signed up.'

'Yeah, I've already lost 5kg since I started my workplace challenge', I grinned.

'Good on you!' said Phil. 'You're doing so well!'

I felt an extra bounce in my step as I made my way to the circuit. My confidence and attitude had already begun to improve, and getting positive affirmations from others gave me even more motivation to keep pushing forward.

A week later, I had a coaching call with my mindset coach, Charlotte. 'For the first time in years, I'm finally starting to feel happy about myself and where my life is heading', I told her. 'I've been able to go several weeks without eating fatty foods or sugar. The other day, when my parents offered me steak, I said no, and it was a pretty easy decision for me. I'm finally losing weight and keeping it off.'

'That is amazing', said Charlotte. 'You see what is happening, Oliver? You are learning how to love yourself now. You have taken massive action in leading a healthier life, and the results are already showing.'

That coaching session was another turning point for me. It was in that moment that I first understood what self-love really is. For years, I had been filled with self-loathing and self-pity. I had never felt satisfied with the person

I saw in the mirror, and I would often ask myself, 'Who on earth could like me?' My discovery of self-love allowed me to have a clearer vision of who I wanted to be. I was determined to push myself and work even harder to achieve my goals. My results were becoming visible, not just physically, but mentally as well. After a few weeks, I noticed that my energy had improved. It had been a while since I had experienced a major bout of anxiety or depression. I no longer felt like I wanted to end my life. Instead, I was filled with a new zeal for living.

In mid-January, I stopped by Phil's office to say hi before beginning my usual workout. 'Hey, Phil', I said. 'How's it going?'

Phil glanced up, and a surprised look spread across his face. 'Hi, Oliver! Say, can I get you to turn just to your left?'

I wasn't sure of the reason, but I nodded and turned.

'How amazing is that! You're looking slimmer after only a month. Good on you!'

I grinned, looking down at my stomach. He was right. My gut was almost gone. For the first time since my sky dive, I felt extremely proud of myself for what I had achieved.

I had finished my training session and was on my way out to head home for the evening when I had another chat to Phil.

'Hey Oli, have you thought about doing more one-on-one sessions?' he asked.

'Actually, yes. That would help me reach my milestones faster, right?'

'Absolutely. Having a personal trainer will make a huge difference in your progress, and I know just the guy. His name is William. He's amazing.'

'Okay, sure. That sounds great', I replied.

Phil introduced me to William, and we planned to begin our sessions the next day. I was excited to work with a trainer one-on-one. The single session I'd had with Mark had helped me turn my life around, and I knew that regular sessions would make an even bigger impact. I didn't know exactly what I was getting myself into, but I knew that personal training would help me avoid injury. It would also keep me accountable to my fitness objectives. Besides that, I couldn't have anticipated the changes that were about to come.

Towards the end of January, I realised that it had been more than a month since I had accepted the invitation to participate in the Biggest Loser challenge. I weighed myself weekly at the gym, even though I knew it was only one metric of health. Still, it helped me keep track of my progress. With the exception of the week before Christmas, I maintained slow but steady weight loss. Each week, I was losing just over a kilogram. I remembered back to the day I began my gym membership. I had barely been able to get through a ten-minute jog on the treadmill. Not even two months later, I could run continuously for ten minutes and finish off with a two-minute sprint with a pace of 17km/h. Of course, I would be out of breath by the time I completed my workout, but now I felt exhilarated instead of exhausted.

William and I worked several days a week on circuit training, rotating between arms, legs, and back. At the beginning of February, I arrived at the gym for leg day and warmed up before my session.

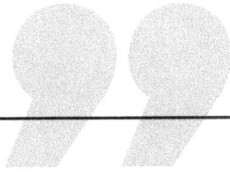

I REMEMBERED BACK TO THE DAY I BEGAN MY GYM MEMBERSHIP. I HAD BARELY BEEN ABLE TO GET THROUGH A TEN-MINUTE JOG ON THE TREADMILL. NOT EVEN TWO MONTHS LATER, I COULD RUN CONTINUOUSLY FOR TEN MINUTES AND FINISH OFF WITH A TWO-MINUTE SPRINT WITH A PACE OF 17KM/H. OF COURSE, I WOULD BE OUT OF BREATH BY THE TIME I COMPLETED MY WORKOUT, BUT NOW I FELT EXHILARATED INSTEAD OF EXHAUSTED.

'Okay, are you ready to start?' asked William as I finished my jog on the treadmill.

'All good to go!' I replied.

William led me to the leg extension machine and raised the weight to 40kg. The exercise didn't feel all that difficult at the start, but I wondered if I was getting the technique right.

'Okay, what I want you to do is to raise, hold for three seconds, and then slowly lower your legs', said William.

I nodded. I realised that I had not been holding my extended position for long enough, which did not allow my quads to extend properly. As soon as I started executing the exercise properly, the cramps began to kick in.

'This isn't going to get any easier, is it?' I grimaced.

'Nope!' smiled William. 'But you're going to get through it!'

After completing three sets of twelve repetitions, we moved to leg curls, and of course, I struggled with this exercise as well. By the time I reached the third set, my legs were shaking. We moved to the squat machine, and after three more sets, I finally felt my legs giving out on me. Learning these new, unfamiliar techniques was a struggle, but I knew that it would allow me to reach my next fitness milestone.

William must have read my mind. 'You know, each set you do is going to bring you closer to your long-term objectives.'

'Yes, I'm looking forward to it! I want to improve my health, and I want to lose more weight. I have lost nearly 10kg since December. Here, do you want to see?' I asked as I pulled out my phone to show William my 'before' and 'after' photos.

'Geez!' said William in absolute disbelief. In the 'before' photo, I had the beginnings of a beer belly. Now, my stomach had muscular definition.

'Oliver, could you please text me these photos?' asked William. 'If it's okay with you, I want to share this on my Instagram. Man, your transformation so far is amazing. Probably the best I have seen so far at this gym.'

'Not a problem', I said as I sent him the photos. It was a true compliment to know that my trainer wanted to share my results with his Instagram followers.

When you make the decision to change, whether it's kicking an unhealthy habit, losing weight, or improving your overall health, your action plan will become clearer once you define your end goal. Ask yourself this question: 'What is my *Why*?' *Why* do you want to make this change, and *why* do you want to do it *now*? When you have a detailed understanding of this goal, your transformation will become easier. Once you determine your objective, take note of your action plans, and make sure they are achievable. As you focus your mind and train your body to engage in these new patterns, you will build healthy habits that will last a lifetime.

05

TIME TO FACE NEW CHALLENGES

At some point in our life, we must accept that it is up to us to face the challenges that lie before us and push through to the other side. Before I began my journey, I was trapped in a shrinking world of anxiety. I would commit to an event or social occasion, only to back out at the last minute. I thought that no one would ever like me, and I was too afraid to question my limiting beliefs. When I would arrive at a challenge, I would listen to negative people who told me that it was too hard or too risky. Instead of building myself up, I would convince myself that I would never be able to reach my goals.

In January of 2018, I decided to reward my recent self-development work with a weekend away in Canberra to visit my friend, Di. I was introduced to Di through mutual friends on Facebook, but we had never gotten to meet in real life. I was excited to finally spend some time with my friend in person.

A few days before I was due to leave, Di texted me. 'Hey Oliver, I was thinking that we could go on a daytrip and take a hike up Mount Kosciuszko. It will be a long day, and it's going to push us to our limits, but I know it'll be a lot of fun. What do you think?'

'That actually sounds like something I'd like to try', I texted her back. 'These days, I'm all about testing my limits.'

'Perfect. The hike opens at 9:00 a.m., and it's about a three-hour drive, so we'll need to leave the house at around 5:30 a.m.'

'Sounds good! Let's do it!'

Over the first few weeks of my transformation, I discovered the importance of taking risks. Even if I didn't meet my goals right away, I didn't allow myself to give up. I learned that failure isn't an excuse to quit; instead, it is an opportunity to improve. Each time I fell down, I got back up and did a better job the next time. It turned out that failing repeatedly was the key to my success. Through adversity, I learned that you will only find out how much you are capable of by saying 'yes' to challenging yourself.

It was the morning of Australia Day, and I was finishing my last-minute packing before making my way to the airport for my flight to Canberra. Once I had everything organised in my suitcase, I drove to Rohit's house. He was kind enough to let me leave my car there over the weekend so I wouldn't have to pay for airport parking. I felt blessed to have such good friends in my life.

After a twenty-minute ride, Rohit dropped me off just outside Terminal 1 at Melbourne Airport. I arrived at my gate in time for boarding and looked outside to see an ATR 72 aircraft waiting at the stand. I had booked with Virgin Australia, and I decided to treat myself to an upgrade to Business Class. We boarded the plane, and I searched for my seat. As is common for ATR aeroplanes, Business Class was located at the rear of the aircraft. Finally, I found my window seat, and I glanced outside in excitement at the turboprop engines ahead of me. Even though it would only be a one-hour flight, it would still be a joy to watch the engines in action.

Before I knew it, we were ascending into the clouds. It was a stormy day, and the turbulent air jostled the aeroplane as we flew north to Canberra. Still, I was not concerned, even when the plane hit a particularly rough patch of air. Several of the passengers around me gasped as we lost a few hundred metres of altitude, but I kept my cool. I looked out at the turboprop engine on my side of the plane, knowing that it would get us safely to our destination. After about a half hour at cruising altitude, we began our descent towards Canberra Airport.

We arrived at our gate five minutes after touching down. I disembarked as quickly as possible, given that my seat was at the back of the plane, and I powerwalked my way to baggage claim. As I descended the escalator, I saw Di standing by my flight's baggage carousel, waving at me with both arms. I waved right back, grinning broadly. I felt somewhat nervous for our hike the next day, but excitement outweighed my fear.

'You look fantastic!' said Di as she opened her arms to give me a hug.

'Thank you so much!' I replied. 'Such a pleasure to meet you in person, Di.'

'I barely recognised you from your old photos when you came down the stairs', said Di.

'Yeah, I was starting to get pretty big', I nodded. 'I'm glad I began my transformation before things got too far out of hand.'

After I collected my luggage, we climbed in Di's car and made our way to the city centre. We decided to dine at a sushi restaurant as Di knew that I was excluding meat from my diet. After a delicious meal of salmon sashimi, we drove to Di's house and got ready for an early start the next day. We would have to leave for our hike before sunrise. After briefly saying hello to Di's dog, a friendly Staffy named Phoenix, I showered and got ready for bed. Di's office doubled as a guest bedroom, and her convertible sofa was surprisingly comfortable. No sooner had I climbed under the covers than I was fast asleep.

The next morning, I awoke at 5:00 a.m. and prepared myself for the three-hour trip to Mount Kosciuszko. Di packed us water and snacks, and we each brought an extra change of clothes in case we got caught in the rain. Phoenix bounded to the door as we were heading out.

'I don't think she's too happy', said Di. 'I only took her for a quick walk this morning. She'll have to run around in the back yard today. It's okay, darling, I promise we'll have a nice long walk tomorrow. Now, be a good dog.'

We left the house at 5:30 a.m. and headed south on the Monaro Highway towards the New South Wales border. We spent most of the drive engaging in light conversation, allowing the time to go by as we drew closer to our destination. At 9:00 a.m., we arrived at Thredbo Village where we planned to begin our hike.

'I'm just going to get our chairlift passes', said Di as she made her way to the welcome centre.

'Sounds good', I replied. 'You packed our food, so I'll handle beverages. I am going to get myself a coffee. Did you want anything?'

'I would love a hot chocolate', said Di with a smile.

'Sure thing. Be right back.'

I stopped briefly at a café to get our drinks and handed Di her hot chocolate in exchange for my pass. Warm beverages in hand, we made our way to the chairlift that would take us to the start of the trail.

After a scenic ride up the mountain, we climbed off the chair lift and started walking. Ten minutes into our hike, I noticed a sign stating that we were 6km away from the top of Mount Kosciuszko. I felt the blood drain from my face. Something inside of me said, 'That's way too far. I'll never make it.' I shook my head, trying to tell the voice to be quiet. Then another voice told me, 'Oliver, you did not come all this way for nothing. Just keep putting one foot in front of the other. You are going to make it to the top.'

'We've got a bit of a way to go', said Di, nodding at the sign. 'According to our current pace, we should be at the top in approximately an hour and a half. Still, I believe we can do better than that.'

'Yes. I think it's doable', I nodded.

It was at that point that I decided to re-shift my mindset from 'It's not possible' to 'Let's to this'. We continued our hike along the trail, overtaking several groups of tourists who were pausing for a breather. This reminded me of my first session at the gym where I had to stop every few minutes on the treadmill to catch my breath. Now, I was able to keep going at a consistent pace.

'Do you want me to slow down at all?' asked Di.

'No, I can keep up', I replied. I refused to stop. We passed a sign stating that we were 5km from the top of the mountain, but I didn't let the distance faze me. Soon, we arrived at a sign for 4km, then 3km. I looked up, and I could finally see the peak of the mountain ahead of us.

'We're not far off from the top!' said Di. 'The last kilometre or two may be harder as the trail gets steeper. Are you coping okay?'

'Yeah. Let's keep going. I'll see how I do towards the end', I replied, trying not to pant. My quads were beginning to burn slightly but not enough to force me to stop.

I found that the process of hiking had an uplifting effect. Each step I took gave me more energy and more self-belief. Even though I was tired, I kept moving forward. Earlier in my life, I would have let the discomfort defeat me. Now, I was able to keep walking, each step bringing me closer to the summit.

> IT WAS AT THAT POINT THAT I DECIDED TO RE-SHIFT MY MINDSET FROM 'IT'S NOT POSSIBLE' TO 'LET'S TO THIS'

I told myself, 'Oliver, enough is enough. Giving up is not an option'. As I walked, I repeated to myself in my head, 'I'm capable of doing this; I know I can do this'. The more I focussed on the climb, the easier the process became. With each footfall, I felt more confident that I would be able to reach the top. This was a revelation for me. I realised that commitment is a key ingredient to success. When you commit to doing something with every fibre of your being, you dramatically increase your likelihood of achieving your goal.

After what seemed to be a challenging hike at the beginning, I felt a huge sense of accomplishment as we reached the peak of the mountain. 'Amazing! That was actually far easier than I thought!' I exclaimed. 'I'm so glad I didn't psych myself out like I used to.' I grinned at Di as we surveyed the view from the summit. The hilly, green terrain below stretched on for kilometres on end.

'I think that was far too easy for you', laughed Di.

'I completely agree', I nodded.

'I'm just checking our timer', said Di. 'We made it to the top in one hour and five minutes.'

'That's great time', I smiled. 'I'm really happy with that.' We spent a few moments on the top to take some photos and revel in the view.

'Let's have a snack and some water, and then let's head back down, okay?' asked Di.

'Sounds good', I said, munching on a muesli bar. 'I'm ready whenever you are.'

We hiked our way back down the trail and decided to make a few stops along the way to take more photos. I wanted to document the journey as this was my first time summiting any mountain, let alone the tallest mountain in Australia. After an hour, we eventually reached the chairlift that would take us back down to Thredbo Village.

> **I REALISED THAT COMMITMENT IS A KEY INGREDIENT TO SUCCESS. WHEN YOU COMMIT TO DOING SOMETHING WITH EVERY FIBRE OF YOUR BEING, YOU DRAMATICALLY INCREASE YOUR LIKELIHOOD OF ACHIEVING YOUR GOAL.**

'I bet this view of the Village reminds you of your skydive', said Di as we climbed onto the chairlift.

'You know what, it somewhat does', I replied, looking down at the quaint rooftops of Thredbo far below. 'I will never forget that experience. Absolutely incredible.'

We were both hungry after our hike, so we decided to stop for lunch at the Village. 'I think this looks like a good place to chill for a bit', said Di, pointing to a nearby café. 'How are you feeling after the climb?'

'I'm feeling quite good', I said as we sat at an empty table. 'I'm famished, but I don't feel too worn out.'

'You did really well on the trail. Just goes to show how much you are improving', said Di. 'Not sure what you're ordering, but I am going to go for a chicken baguette.'

I looked at the menu. 'I'm just going to have the falafel wrap, I think.'

I walked up to the counter to pay for our food. The falafel tasted heavenly as a post-workout meal. We ate our lunch quickly and then decided to walk a little more before heading back.

'It's really nice and peaceful here at Thredbo', I said. 'I definitely want to come back here again.'

'You should!' said Di. 'You know, it's an awesome ski resort during the winter months.'

'I haven't skied since high school, but I'd like to get back into it', I nodded.

'It's so much fun', grinned Di. 'Just picture this place with lots of snow. You'd love it!'

As we chatted, we made our way back to Di's car. Dark clouds were rolling in, and we didn't want to be caught in the rain. Soon, we were on our way back to Canberra. Most of the drive was spent in silence. Exhaustion was setting in, and we both needed to focus on the road. Three hours later, we crossed the border to the Australian Capital Territory.

As we pulled up to Di's house, we could see Phoenix peering out the front window, her tail waggling her entire body with joy. She greeted us as we walked in the front door, and we all made our way to the back yard. Di stopped in the kitchen to fetch us glasses of ice water, and we settled in her sun loungers, relaxing after the long day. As I sipped my glass of water, Phoenix decided to jump up on my lap.

'Oh lord!' said Di. 'Sorry about that! She does that whenever someone's not paying attention.' She got up and tried to wrestle the dog off my lap.

'No dramas', I said. 'She can stay. You know, I used to be terrified of dogs when I was a kid, but now I rather like them. At least the friendly ones. Phoenix is a good dog.'

'Suit yourself', laughed Di. 'When you stand up, she'll get off. I'm going to start cooking dinner. I'm grilling us salmon steaks since I know you don't eat meat.'

As Di prepared the barbeque for our meal, her teenage son came to the back yard to greet us.

'Oliver, please meet my son, Brayden.'

'Pleasure to meet you', I said.

'You too', replied Brayden. 'Thanks for coming to visit mum and me.'

Di finished cooking our dinner, and I got up to help her set the backyard picnic table. Phoenix made a whining sound when I stood up, but she didn't protest otherwise. Di, Brayden, and I all gathered round to help ourselves to salmon and salad.

'Dobar tek', I said as we sat down to eat. Di is Croatian, too, so I knew that she and Brayden would understand this common saying for 'Good appetite'.

'Dobar tek', replied Di and Brayden in unison, raising their glasses with a smile.

We ate in silence. Di and I were both tired, and we didn't have much energy for conversation. After dinner, I took a shower and felt somewhat refreshed. At least, I no longer felt like I was about to fall asleep at any moment. As I settled in for the evening, I made my way to the lounge room and engaged in conversation with Di and Brayden. Phoenix came over and looked at me, whining softly. I tapped my palm on the couch, allowing her to jump up on my lap.

'Look at that', smiled Di. 'She's a happy girl. She really knows how to turn on the charm when she wants to.'

'I wonder if she can tell that I used to be afraid of dogs. Maybe she's trying to make sure that I feel comfortable around her.' I started lightly scratching Phoenix behind her left ear, and she rested her head more towards my palm.

'Oh, she's not going to want you to leave now', laughed Di.

It was close to 10:00 p.m., and all I could think about was the comfortable bed in the guest room. I said goodnight to everyone and gave Phoenix a final pat on the head. I made my way to my room and fell asleep almost as soon as my head hit the pillow.

I woke up the following morning at 6:00 a.m., feeling refreshed after a solid eight hours of sleep. I opened the bedroom door and was immediately greeted by a waggly Phoenix.

'Phoenix, down!' shouted Di. 'Morning, Oliver. Did you sleep well?'

'Morning, Di. Slept like a log', I replied.

'I'll take the dog for a walk in a few minutes', said Di. 'You can come if you like.'

'Perfect, I'll get ready', I nodded, walking back to my room to dress quickly.

'Shall we go for a walk, Phoenix?' asked Di as she picked up the leash. Phoenix jumped up and down in excitement. Soon, the three of us were walking out the front door and making our way to the local primary school. 'She always loves to run around here chasing rabbits', laughed Di. We completed a walk around the schoolyard while Phoenix sprinted ahead of us, looking for rabbits to chase. After a half hour, we made our way back to Di's house. She prepared us a breakfast of scrambled eggs, sourdough toast, and coffee.

'C'mon', said Di, leading the way to the back yard. 'Let's have breakfast outside. The weather is perfect this morning.'

After we finished our meal, I went to the guest room to pack my suitcase for my flight back to Melbourne that evening. Then we climbed in Di's car to do more sightseeing. We went to the National Arboretum Canberra before heading to the Old Parliament House, the art museum, and the Telstra Tower. We ordered a light lunch from a café nearby and had a picnic down by Lake Burley Griffin. The sun made its way across the sky, and soon it was past its zenith.

'Well, I guess we should start heading to the airport', said Di, checking the time on her phone.

I glanced at my watch. It was 2:00 p.m., and I needed to be at the terminal in an hour. Luckily, it was only a twenty-minute ride to the airport from here. 'You're right', I nodded. 'The time sure has flown.'

We climbed in Di's car, and we were at the departure level before we knew it.

'Di, thank you so much for looking after me and showing me around', I said.

'Oliver, it was my absolute pleasure', Di replied as she reached out her arms to give me a hug. 'Come back any time. I'd love to take you skiing at Thredbo Village. It will be fun!'

'Thanks so much for being such a good friend, Di', I said, hugging her back. 'I will absolutely take you up on that offer.'

I headed into the terminal and dropped off my suitcase at the check-in counter. The attendant gave me my boarding pass and told me my gate

"

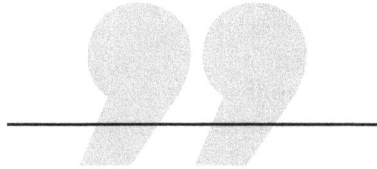

IF YOU ARE OFFERED AN
OPPORTUNITY TO TEST
YOURSELF, DON'T BE
AFRAID TO RISE TO THE
CHALLENGE. IF YOU FAIL,
DON'T GIVE UP; FAILURE
GIVES YOU ANOTHER
CHANCE TO IMPROVE AND
RISE UP AGAIN.

---

number. Then I made my way through security and headed to the Virgin Australia lounge as I was travelling Business Class back to Melbourne. I texted Rohit to let him know that the flight was on time.

'See you soon, bro', came his swift reply. 'Just so you know, it's hot here, so be prepared!' The minutes marched by, and soon it was time to board. I settled into my window seat up front with the seat next to me unoccupied. We departed for Melbourne on schedule at 5:00 p.m., and I enjoyed a meal of hummus and flat bread inflight with a glass of shiraz. I smiled at the perks of flying Business Class, acknowledging the importance of treating myself to a little luxury now and then.

We landed in Melbourne just after 6:00 p.m., and I was greeted by a 39-degree heatwave. I waited ten minutes after collecting my luggage before Rohit came to pick me up.

'Bro, you were right when you said it was hot today', I exclaimed as I climbed into Rohit's car.

'Mate, it is boiling here!' he laughed. 'So how was your trip?'

'It was beautiful. I Hiked Mount Kosciuszko yesterday morning, and I did some sightseeing in Canberra this afternoon. I still can't believe that I climbed to the top of the tallest mountain in Australia.'

'You're getting strong, mate!' he said. 'Good for you!'

I stayed at Rohit's house for half an hour for some cold fruits and water before I made my way back home. I decided to go easy on myself the next day, so I took the day off work and didn't go to the gym. Still, I was no worse for wear. I looked in the mirror and grinned at myself. The man who grinned back at me looked healthy and fit. 'Good work, Oliver. You're doing great', I said to the mirror, and I smiled as my reflection mouthed the affirmation back to me.

When we encounter a task that we deem to be challenging, part of us will often say 'no' because we see it as 'too hard'. When I agreed to hike up Mount Kosciuszko, it was important for me to confront this limiting belief. I needed to prove to myself that it was possible and that I could do it. If you are offered an opportunity to test yourself, don't be afraid to rise to the challenge. If you fail, don't give up; failure gives you another chance to improve and rise up again. You have what it takes to grow, and you will be able to overcome the hurdles before you; all you need is preparation and the drive to step out of your comfort zone. Once you succeed, you will realise that you can do nearly anything if you make up your mind to accomplish it.

06

MY JOURNEY TO
SUCCESS

No matter what journey you are on, it is worth sharing it with your friends. When you do, you will encourage them along their own path of self-development. There will be obstacles along the way; after all, this is never designed to be easy. But no matter how challenging the journey may seem, don't give up. By showing that you are willing to do what it takes to achieve your goal, you will lead others by example. It all starts with you making the decision to say yes to the challenges that lie ahead. The greatest adversity often leads to the greatest achievements.

In 2018, I found out that my friend Shilpa was finalist in the Australia Galaxy Pageant. She had competed in another pageant the year before, and she had won a prize. That gave her the confidence to try out for this larger pageant. In order to prepare for her audition, she went through an extensive workout routine. I felt a kinship with her as we both worked to transform ourselves towards our goals.

One day, I noticed several posts on Facebook regarding the upcoming pageant. Her parents, Rohit and Shalini, were thrilled that Shilpa had been selected as a finalist, and they were announcing their plans to fly to the Gold Coast, where the competition would be held. Right then, I knew that I wanted to be there in person, too, so I could support my friend. The next morning, I requested a few days off from work, and to my delight, my manager granted my request.

I could barely contain my excitement as I messaged Rohit and Shalini. 'Just wanted to let you know that I got an approval for time off work, and I would love to support Shilpa in person!'

'Oliver, that would mean so much to us. Of course, we would love for you to be there', came Shalini's swift reply.

I didn't waste any time in booking my flights and accommodation. I would arrive before the pageant and spend a few days hanging out with Rohit and his family. I couldn't wait.

On the day of my flight, I left the multi-level carpark in Docklands after a gruelling session at the gym. I was still sweating as I drove out and made my way to the airport. I had spare time when I arrived at Tullamarine and decided to park at the aircraft viewing area until I was able to check my luggage in. After an hour, I left my car at the long-term carpark and made my way to Terminal Four. Check in was easy as I printed out the tag for my suitcase and made my way through security.

As I approached my gate, I looked out at the large Jetstar A321 that was going to take me and my fellow passengers to Coolangatta.

'Are you heading to the Gold Coast for a holiday?' asked the gate attendant as I checked the status of my flight.

'Sort of', I replied. 'I'll be there to support a friend who's a finalist for a beauty pageant. But I'll make sure to find a few days to relax.'

'That definitely sounds like a lot of fun', smiled the agent.

'Yeah. To be honest, I haven't given myself a decent break for the last five months', I sighed.

'Oh, been working hard, I take it?' asked the agent, raising her eyebrows.

'Not just at work but on myself as well', I replied. 'I decided to turn my life around and start a journey to better health. I have lost 20kg since December.' I took out my phone to show her my before and after photos.

'Oh, wow. That is incredible', she said, peering over her desk. 'Good on you!'

'Thank you. I'm definitely not going back to the person who I was once upon a time.'

It wasn't long before the gateway doors opened, and I made my way to board my flight. I'd strategically chosen a seat near the back of the aircraft, just behind the wing. It would give me the best view of the engines as they roared to life, propelling us on our two-hour journey.

Before I knew it, we began our descent into Coolangatta. I peered out the window, watching as the New South Wales countryside gave way to the Queensland coast. We touched down at ten minutes ahead of schedule and taxied to our gate. I was no doubt the only one on board who wished the beautiful flight had been longer.

I arrived at my hotel and skyped with Charlotte, my coach, for our regular check-in. I told Charlotte about my conversation with the gate agent earlier in the day. 'She seemed really interested in my story. I think I'm at the point where I'm ready to share my journey with others more. I think I can encourage them to change for the better.'

'You are doing so well with your transformation', said Charlotte. 'So many people give up within the first month, but you said yes on committing to a better you, and there are no signs of you stopping. You know, I have an idea. Why don't you create a page on Facebook and Instagram purely on the journey you have been on since December?'

'To be honest, I hadn't really considered documenting things on social media', I replied, 'but I am definitely ready to share my journey.'

'Yeah. It would be so good to set up a page to share your progress', said Charlotte. 'You could call it "My journey to success".'

I nodded. 'That's a great idea. I think I'll use my time here to create my page and start bringing in my audience. Plus, that will let me use my down time here productively. I'm actually excited to begin!'

I woke up the next morning and went to meet up with Rohit, Shalini, and Shilpa at the Marriott where they were staying. When I arrived, they were sitting together in the hotel lobby. It looked like they were getting ready to head off for the day.

'Hey Rohit!' I called. 'Great to see you, mate!'

'Oliver! Good to see you here in the Gold Coast!' said Rohit as he reached out to shake my hand.

'Yes!' said Shilpa. 'Great to see you! Thank you so much for flying up all the way to support me!'

'It is my absolute pleasure to be here', I smiled, nodding to Shilpa. 'Besides, it'll give us all a chance to relax for a few days.'

'Well, I've got to go to a pageant photoshoot up on the second level', said Shilpa, 'but I'll see everyone later!' She hugged her parents and shook my hand, and then she rushed off to the elevators.

A few minutes later, Rohit and Shalini headed out to the airport to pick up Shalini's parents, Hari and Pushpa. Soon, the whole family would be there to cheer Shilpa on.

I went out for a stroll on the hotel grounds and found a nice spot of shade where I could start building my Facebook page. It didn't take me long to come up with the name. I called it 'Oliver's Journey to Success'. That would remind me of my success goals, and it would keep me focussed on the transformative path I was taking. I decided to use the same title for my Instagram, and I linked it to my newly created Facebook page.

The hours passed quickly, and before I knew it, Rohit and Shalini had arrived with Hari and Pushpa. Shilpa returned from her photoshoot soon after, and we all went to hang out by the pool.

'Now this is what we call a relaxing time out, mate', said Rohit. 'We've all earned a bit of vacation.'

'I definitely needed this', I nodded. 'I've been working too hard lately. I think it was time that I took a break.'

'If you're not doing anything tonight, you're welcome to join us for an event that the pageant is having', said Rohit.

'That sounds great, mate', I said. 'I think I'll head back to my hotel and get ready then. See you this evening!'

I returned to my apartment and continued working on the contents for my Facebook page. It was going to take some time to finish it, but I gave myself a metaphorical pat on the back for getting started. 'Good onya, Oliver', I said to myself. 'The first step is always the hardest.'

I uploaded the 'before' photos I'd taken when I started my journey back in November. Then I stood in front of the mirror and took a few selfies to upload as my 'current' photos. As I stared at my reflection, I compared it to the pictures I'd taken only a few months ago. It was a proud moment for me, and it gave me the hunger to keep progressing with my journey.

I opened my Messenger and sent Charlotte a quick text. 'You'll be please to know that I've created a page for myself on FB and Insta! It's called "Oliver's Journey to Success". Please have a look!'

'Brilliant!' Charlotte texted back. 'You are taking massive action, and I love it. You are definitely walking your talk, and I couldn't be prouder of you.'

I changed into a smart outfit and walked back to the Marriott to meet up with Rohit's family. We all made our way up to the ballroom on the second level for a social event. We milled about the room for a while, and then we saw that a few of the previous pageant winners were meeting the guests. I went over and got selfies with a few of them. Afterwards, I marvelled at my courage. There was no way I would have felt comfortable asking a beauty pageant winner for a selfie a few months ago.

After a half hour of this, I started to get sleepy. I had reached my social saturation point. I turned to Rohit and said, 'I might call it an evening and get something to eat on the way back. It's getting late.'

'You're not going to stay for the rest of the evening?' asked Rohit.

'No, I'm getting a bit tired, and I still need to do some work tonight', I replied.

'No worries, mate. I'll see you tomorrow.'

As I made my way back to my hotel, I took a detour to pick up a meal from a nearby Thai restaurant. Even though I was on vacation, I was determined to keep up my pescatarian diet as much as possible.

The next day was the evening of the pageant finals. Rohit and I spent the afternoon together, exploring the downtown. We stopped at a Korean restaurant for lunch, which gave me another opportunity to maintain my diet. Rohit ordered Korean fried chicken, while I chose spicy seafood with noodles.

'Is that too hot for you, mate?' grinned Rohit as he noticed that I was starting to sweat.

'I can actually handle the heat. This is just how I react to eating spicy food', I laughed.

We spent the remaining afternoon chatting about AIFAV's upcoming events for the year. Soon, it was time to go to the event hall. I sat in the front row with Rohit, Shalini, Hari, and Pushpa.

> THERE WILL BE OBSTACLES ALONG THE WAY; AFTER ALL, THIS IS NEVER DESIGNED TO BE EASY. BUT NO MATTER HOW CHALLENGING THE JOURNEY MAY SEEM, DON'T GIVE UP. BY SHOWING THAT YOU ARE WILLING TO DO WHAT IT TAKES TO ACHIEVE YOUR GOAL, YOU WILL LEAD OTHERS BY EXAMPLE.

Soon, the moment we had all been waiting for arrived. Shilpa's name was called, and she glided onto the stage. The five of us gasped with admiration. You see, Shilpa was born with mild cerebral palsy. When she was a baby, the doctors had told her parents that she would never be able to walk. Every step that she took across the stage proved to everyone that she had beat the odds.

Shalini soared through the pageant. It was inspiring to see her radiate confidence as she strutted along with the other women. All the hard work and physical therapy that she'd endured had paid off. I remember looking over at Rohit and Shalini, and their eyes were shining with tears of pride. We all let out a collective cheer as Shilpa was awarded the prize for the Eco Friendly Category. I was so happy for her. It felt almost magical to watch someone that I cared about accomplish such a big goal. Once the pageant came to a close, we all went backstage to congratulate Shilpa. Her parents and grandparents were ecstatic as they rushed over to hug her.

'You did amazing out there, Shilpa', I smiled as I reached down to give her a hug. 'We're all so proud of you.'

'Thank you, Oliver', she beamed. 'I'm so glad you could be here! This has been one of the most amazing nights of my life.'

If you are on a journey to better health, you might ask yourself whether it is worth it to share it with others. I can assure you that it is. When you bring other people along with you, it gives them hope and inspiration that they, too, can achieve what they have set their mind to accomplish. Putting yourself out there can feel like a big risk at times, but when you see how much your story touches other people's lives, it vindicates every step you've taken along the way.

WALKING A BALANCED PATH

As you work hard to get into shape and focus on new health goals, your knowledge in fitness gets tested as well. Over time, you get so used to the routine that you tend to explore each exercise to the finest of details. It is easy to pick up the right techniques from how you are positioned to how you breathe during each exercise. Your support staff will test you—everyone from your trainer to your doctor—not just to ensure that you are improving, but also to ensure that they are doing their part in helping you succeed.

The middle of autumn was fast approaching, and I maintained my routine of training five days a week, as I'd promised myself earlier in the year. It got to a point where I had programmed myself to train consistently. Every day after work, my feet carried me as if on autopilot to the Anytime Fitness gym.

One day, I got a text from my trainer, William, telling me that he had an opening for an extra training session on Saturdays. I jumped at the chance. I knew what I was getting myself into by committing to training six days per week. It was going to require not only hard work, but also dedication in keeping myself committed. I was more focussed on my goals than ever, and just the thought of that fuelled my determination to succeed.

I made my way to Anytime Fitness Collins Square on a quiet Saturday morning, ready to begin my one-on-one session with William. It was a strange feeling coming to the Docklands on a quiet Saturday morning; the normally bustling office complex felt almost deserted. I went in and got changed to my training gear before warming up on the treadmill.

> **YOUR SUPPORT STAFF WILL TEST YOU EVERYONE FROM YOUR TRAINER TO YOUR DOCTORNOT JUST TO ENSURE THAT YOU ARE IMPROVING, BUT ALSO TO ENSURE THAT THEY ARE DOING THEIR PART IN HELPING YOU SUCCEED.**

William walked into the gym ready for my session. 'Hey Oli, are we ready to go?' he asked as he came up to me to shake my hand.

'Let's do this', I replied. 'What are we training today?'

'Back and biceps', said William. 'It's gonna be an intense session, so get ready!'

William led me over to the lat pulldown machine. I completed three sets at 42kg, and then we moved onto bicep curls.

'It would be good to work more on strengthening your shoulders as well', said William.

'Always room for improvement', I nodded. 'I'll do whatever it takes to hit my goals. Let's go!'

We moved on to lateral raises to work my shoulders and reached 32kg by the second set.

'Man, you're getting stronger!' said William. 'Good onya!'

'Thanks, man', I smiled. 'I've been testing myself to see how far I can go, and if I have room to increase the weights.'

'Yeah, what you're doing is definitely working', nodded William. 'I'm happy with your progress.'

'Good! Though there's still room to improve', I said.

'One hundred percent, man. You never stop learning or growing', said William, clapping me on the back.

I finished another set on lateral raises, and William reached out to shake my hand, indicating that the session was finished. I felt proud that

I had accomplished six days of training that week. Now all I had to do was keep up this workout routine. I didn't know at the time that this would be more difficult than I'd anticipated.

Over the course of that autumn, I started to feel more lethargic than usual. I was not sure whether I was feeling run down, coming down with a cold, or just getting burnt out. I put in an effort during my gym sessions, but every time I went to work out, I felt like I had been drained of energy.

I knew that something wasn't right.

As I finished my session one day, I stopped by to have a chat to Carla, the assistant manager.

'Hey Oliver, how did you go?' asked Carla.

'To be honest, I didn't go as well as I hoped', I said, shaking my head. 'I've been feeling run down lately, and I think it showed in my performance today.'

'You've been off meat for a little while, haven't you?' she asked.

'Since last December', I replied. 'I've only had meat about five times between then and now.'

'It might be worthwhile to see a doctor and get your iron levels checked', said Carla. 'Especially since you haven't had meat for this long. Plus, if you get a full blood panel, you can use it as a metric for monitoring your progress.'

'I hadn't even thought about my iron levels', I confessed. 'I should probably have checked with a doctor before I started my diet. I'll call to make an appointment.'

The following week I went to the Casey Medical Centre to have my blood drawn. A few days later, a nurse called to ask me to come in as soon as possible. My GP, Dr. Morrison, wanted to see me in person to read the results. This made my stomach clench with nervousness. I scheduled the earliest appointment I could, which was early the following Monday. I spent an anxious weekend imagining the worst. The black cloud of depression from my youth began to rear its ugly head. I had to remind myself to take deep breaths and quiet my racing mind. 'It's going to be okay, Oliver', I told myself. 'Don't jump to conclusions. It's all going to turn out fine.'

The next Monday, I took the afternoon off work and went to see my doctor. After a tense half-hour wait, Dr. Morrison finally stepped out into the waiting room.

'Hi Oliver, please come on through.'

I walked into Dr. Morrison's office and asked him, 'Is there any indication of what's wrong? I hope it's not too serious.'

'Well, Oliver, first of all, I wanted to thank you for coming in so quickly', said Dr. Morrison. 'We got your test results back. To start off with, your iron levels are fine. Your cholesterol is a bit high, but not too far off from a normal level.'

'Oh, okay. That's good to hear. So, my iron is normal? That's what I was concerned about. I've been on a pescatarian diet, and I've upped my workouts from five days a week to six. I was thinking that maybe it would be

"

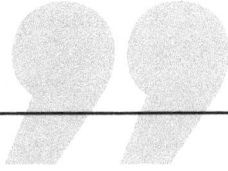

I SPENT AN ANXIOUS
WEEKEND IMAGINING
THE WORST. THE BLACK
CLOUD OF DEPRESSION
FROM MY YOUTH BEGAN
TO REAR ITS UGLY HEAD.
I HAD TO REMIND MYSELF
TO TAKE DEEP BREATHS
AND QUIET MY RACING
MIND. 'IT'S GOING TO BE
OKAY, OLIVER', I TOLD
MYSELF. 'DON'T JUMP TO
CONCLUSIONS. IT'S ALL
GOING TO TURN OUT FINE.'

a good idea to reintroduce meat into my diet. Maybe that would increase my energy? I guess I'm just not sure what's wrong.'

'The only concern we have is that you have a fatty liver. This can be caused by a poor diet in the past, but the good news is that it's reversible.'

'That's...surprising', I said. 'I'm honestly kind of shocked. I cut fatty foods and sugars from my diet a while ago.'

'Well, we don't have consistent records as this is your first full blood panel in several years', said the doctor. 'As you know, it's always best to visit your doctor when you decide to make a lifestyle change, like starting a diet or exercise program. It allows us to establish a baseline that you can measure from. But it is possible that you were headed towards fatty liver disease before you began your healthy lifestyle changes last year. We will need to keep track of your levels from now on, but I think that you will see improvements, so long as you continue to make healthy choices.'

> YOUR SUPPORT STAFF WILL TEST YOU EVERYONE FROM YOUR TRAINER TO YOUR DOCTORNOT JUST TO ENSURE THAT YOU ARE IMPROVING, BUT ALSO TO ENSURE THAT THEY ARE DOING THEIR PART IN HELPING YOU SUCCEED.

'Wow', I said, feeling stunned. 'So, all the junk food I was eating before might have been affecting my liver?'

'We don't have the tests to say that conclusively, but I would say it's quite possible.'

'So, I can use my blood levels as a way to keep track of the effects of my wellness program?'

'Yes. That's a good way to monitor your health. Weight isn't the only metric you should be paying attention to. Your cholesterol and liver function are also important to keep track of.'

'And do you think I'll be able to reduce my fatty liver?'

'That's why we need to keep careful track of your health.'

'So, what do you think about me adding meat to my diet, now that I know my iron levels are okay?'

'I think it's alright in moderation', said the doctor. 'It's important not to have an "all or nothing" mentality about your health. That tends to lead to burnout. And if I had to guess, a reason why you've been feeling fatigued recently may be that you are overtraining. It's better to train moderately and stick with the program than to train to the point of exhaustion and give up.'

'That makes sense', I nodded.

'Oliver, can I ask, when was the last time you had a burger or a cheat meal?'

'Not since I started my training routine last year', I replied.

'Okay', said the doctor. 'I would recommend taking a break from your diet every now and then to maintain balance. Schedule in a healthy cheat meal that you enjoy once a week.'

'I haven't had a burger in ages, and I wouldn't mind getting one', I said.

'I'd say you've earned it. It's clear you've done a great job trimming back. My advice is to keep progressing with your diet and avoid fatty foods and sugars as much as possible, but you can't be strict with your meals 100% of the time. Once you find that balance in your exercise program, I think you will find that your fatigue starts to diminish.'

'Okay. That sounds doable. Thank you so much, Dr. Morrison!'

'You're welcome, Oliver. We'll see you back here soon to monitor your levels.'

I left the doctor's office feeling relieved. My body had recognised that there was something wrong, and I'd listened to that intuition. What's more, I had taken action. I felt proud of myself.

I thought about the doctor's advice, and I could practically taste the burger that I wanted to order. I knew right where to go, too. A few days later, I went to the Balwyn Canteen to visit an old friend—the well-known Melbourne chef and restauranteur, Didier. His restaurant was not far from where I lived, and I used to visit it all the time before I started my diet and exercise regimen. He was always fun to chat to, and his burgers were the best around. I had to admit, I felt a slight pang of guilt as I walked towards the burger joint. I'd gotten so used to eating clean. Still, I told myself, 'Treat yourself, Oliver. You've earned it after all the hard work you've done.'

Didier spotted me as soon as I walked through the restaurant door. 'Oliver!' he exclaimed. 'I haven't seen you in ages. How are you?'

'I've been great. Been working hard over the last few months.'

'I know, mate! I've been watching your progress on Facebook. You're doing awesome!' Didier reached over the counter to shake my hand.

'Thanks, mate. I really appreciate it', I said.

Didier's wife, Adela, came out from the kitchen when she heard my name. She was the manager and helped Didier with the day-to-day running of the Balwyn Canteen.

'Hi Oliver. Long time, no see!' said Adela.

'I know. It's been a few months', I replied.

'It has, and I can see that you have lost some weight', said Adela. 'Good onya! What's your secret?'

'I hope you haven't been starving yourself', joked Didier.

'No, not at all', I chuckled. 'Just altered my diet, and I've been exercising a lot more. I've cut out sugar and fat and replaced it with alkaline foods.'

'Well, whatever you're doing, it's working', said Didier. 'Though, I have to say, you might have wandered into the wrong establishment if you want to avoid sugar and fat!'

'I've actually come here on professional advice', I laughed. 'I've been told I need to have a cheat meal once a week.'

'Well, in that case, you're in the right place!' said Didier. 'Do you know what you'd like to order?'

'I think I'll go for the Senior Burger', I replied.

'Good choice', said Didier as he began to prepare my order.

As Didier brought me my burger, I took some time to appreciate how far I had come. The feeling of guilt left as soon as I took my first bite. My first cheat meal was a smashing success.

'That was quick', said Didier as I finished my meal.

'Yeah, I was pretty hungry', I laughed.

'I bet! How was it?' asked Didier.

'I really enjoyed it.'

'Yeah, I reckon you would have, after being on a strict diet for so long', smiled Didier. 'Good onya for having a cheat meal, Oli. It's well deserved.'

It is important to build rapport and develop a good relationship with your doctor and your personal trainer as they are there not only to help you with your journey, but also to witness it. Diet and exercise are the main components of better health, but it's also essential to visit your doctor and monitor the effects of your workout program. Even if you're worried about the test results you get, they will give you an idea of what you need to do to improve your health. Most of all, though, I encourage you to find balance along your path to wellness. Don't push yourself into an 'all or nothing' approach that will lead to burnout. Instead, have a cheat meal, take a day off, and find ways to enjoy yourself as you grow.

08

STEPPING OUT OF MY COMFORT ZONE

The more you progress on your journey, the further you must step out of your comfort zone. As you move away from that home base, you will probably find it uncomfortable to engage in empowering activities, but you will grow by doing just that. These experiences will make you look back and be glad that you said, 'I can't believe I did that' rather than 'I wish I'd taken the chance'. Once you pass up on an opportunity, you will never know when you will get that offer again.

As autumn turned into winter, I was edging closer towards my fitness goal, not only in losing the weight I wanted to drop, but also in terms of increasing my muscle mass. My self-development brought with it a newfound confidence to participate in opportunities that I would have been afraid to try before. As I was browsing Facebook one day, I noticed a post from Safia, a friend whom I met through AIFAV. Safia was a portrait photographer, and her post announced that she had several new appointments available for headshots. She mostly photographed actors and weddings, but she made herself available to regular people, as well. On several occasions, I had thought about getting a professional photoshoot to document my journey, but I'd never had the confidence to take the leap. This time, however, as I looked at Safia's advertisement, I decided to say 'yes' to the opportunity. I followed the link and booked myself in for a session that weekend.

I woke up early on the day of the shoot, filled with a sense of excitement. I packed my training gear in my gym bag as I was due to have a one-on-one session with William that evening. I got myself prepared, ensuring I was clean shaven, and I put on a nice suit. I arrived at Brimbank Park just before 1:00 p.m. and saw Safia taking out her camera equipment from her car.

'Hey Oliver! Glad to see you here!' said Safia as she reached her arms out to hug me. 'We're just waiting for a few more people to come, and then we'll get started.'

'Are most of the people here for headshots?' I asked.

'Yes, that's right', nodded Safia. 'The people who signed up today are mostly actors and models. They're getting updated headshots for auditions.' Safia looked down at a clipboard with everyone's information. 'Now, you signed up for a photoshoot, but it doesn't say the reason here. Could you tell me a little more about what you'd like to achieve?'

'Well, I'm here to celebrate my weight-loss journey', I said. 'I started a diet and exercise program about a year ago, and I've met a lot of my goals. I've always felt uncomfortable having my picture taken, so I'm challenging myself to do things I'm afraid of. Plus, I want to document my gains.'

'Good for you!' said Safia. 'That's a great reason for a photoshoot. And don't worry, by the way. I'll make sure you're comfortable when I take your picture. It's one of my fortes, if I do say so myself!'

Several more people arrived at the meeting spot in Brimbank Park, and Safia walked over to tell us that she was ready to begin.

'I'll take each of your photos, one person at a time', she said. 'Let's use that tree over there as a background. Now, does anyone want to come first?'

A young man raised his hand. 'I will. I'm Parma.'

'Hi Parma', said Safia, glancing down at her clipboard. 'Are you here for a modelling portfolio?'

'That's right', he said.

'Alright, please stand over here.'

As I watched the photoshoot, I felt a sense of courage come over me. Once Parma was done, I raised my hand to go next.

'Okay, Oliver, if you can stand over here in front of the tree', said Safia as she got her camera ready. 'I'll start by taking a couple of informal shots to get us warmed up.'

I stood and maintained a natural look as Safia took several photos.

'Okay, perfect', she said. 'Now, I'd like you to take your suit jacket off. If you could, please pose, holding your jacket from the collar. I want it to hang down behind your right shoulder. That's right. Okay, now I'd like to get a few photos of you in motion. If you could, please walk towards me, looking out towards the horizon. Keep your eyes forward.'

Safia took several more photos until she made sure that she had some that highlighted my new physique.

After the session, I made my way straight to the Docklands for my one-on-one session with William. I arrived at the gym after a twenty-five-minute drive and proceeded to get changed.

'Oli, how are you?' asked William as I walked towards the treadmill.

'Good to see you, Will. All good and ready to go', I replied as William prepared my session. Today, we would be focusing on chest and triceps.

'How did the photoshoot go?' asked William as I finished my warmup.

'It went great', I replied. 'I actually had a lot of fun.'

'When are you going to get the photos?' asked William.

'Pretty sure within the next day', I said as William handed me a set of weights to work on my triceps. I finished the session and checked my email, but no photos yet.

'Patience, mate', said William. 'You'll get them soon. I can't wait to see!'

Sure enough, I received a message from Safia the following evening, containing five photos from the shoot. A few minutes later, she rang my phone.

'Oliver! Hi! I've just sent you your photos from yesterday, and I wanted to ask you something, if it's okay.'

OF COURSE, SAYING YES WILL EXPOSE YOU TO THINGS THAT ARE OUTSIDE OF YOUR NORM, BUT YOU NEED TO TRUST THE PROCESS. WHEN YOU UNDERGO THIS KIND OF TRANSFORMATION, ALLOW YOURSELF TO LOOK BACK AND CELEBRATE YOUR ACHIEVEMENTS.

'Thank you so much', I replied, looking through the photos. 'I'm really happy with the way they turned out. And sure, what would you like to know?'

'I've been thinking a lot about what we talked about yesterday, about your weight-loss program. I love that you incorporated photography into your journey, and I'd like to write an article about you for my blog. I think this could be a useful milestone for other people who are on a similar journey. Is that okay?'

I was surprised by Safia's request. I didn't realise that my story had touched her to that degree. 'I'd be happy to help you with your article', I said. 'Honestly, I'm flattered.'

'You said that you were on a weight-loss journey. Are there any other struggles you have been through?'

'Well, I was born with a severe language disorder. I struggled mentally for the majority of my 20s. I decided to turn my life around at the end of last year, and so far, I've lost over 20kg.'

'Wow, you are incredible. That's really inspirational, Oliver', said Safia.

'I want to share my story', I replied. 'I was ashamed of my past at first, but I'm too proud to feel like that anymore.'

'I'm so glad you're sharing your story', said Safia. 'I just thought of an idea for a page. I want to call it "Amazing People", and have you first on there.'

'Thank you! That honestly means a lot to me', I said.

'You deserve it', said Safia. 'Okay, give me a few minutes, and I'll write an article about you.'

'I'm really looking forward to seeing it. Thanks again!' I said.

Within twenty minutes, Safia had tagged me in a Facebook post. She had shared five of my photos, and she'd written an article about my struggles and my achievements. I was blown away by how passionate she was in describing my story. The very next day, I was flooded with support from my peers, telling me how inspirational I was. This was a truly proud moment for me.

As the weeks passed, I knew that I was close to celebrating one year since I began my transformation. It allowed me to reflect and look back on my journey that I had embarked on, knowing that there would be more opportunities for me awaiting.

I decided that I wanted to celebrate with the staff at Anytime Fitness as they had been such an integral part of my journey. One morning before work, I went to a nearby winery in Collins Square and ordered a gift that I could pick up later. When I arrived at the gym for my training session that afternoon, I saw Phil in the manager's office.

'Hey matey, how are you?' asked Phil.

'I'm doing really well', I said. 'Are you going anywhere now? I have something to give to you.'

'No, I'll be right here', said Phil.

I walked to the winery and came back shortly after with a bottle of champagne in a gift bag.

'OH MY GOD!' yelled Phil as he saw me coming in.

'Just a small Christmas gift to say thank you for the past year', I replied.

'Oliver, thank you! How kind! You didn't have to do that', said Phil. 'Honestly, your journey over the past year is one of the best that I have seen since I started working in fitness.'

'Wow! Thank you!' I said. 'And please, this is just a small token of the gratitude I feel. It has been about a year since I first signed up here, and my life has totally changed for the better.'

'I remember when you first came in. You are a completely different person now', said Phil. 'Not just with the physical transformation, but your confidence has grown as well.'

'I really had a lack of confidence back then, didn't I?' I chuckled.

'You were definitely shy when you first came in', nodded Phil. 'We have watched you grow over the past year, and we couldn't be any prouder.'

'I'm definitely proud of myself for not only taking the initial step, but for all that I have achieved in just twelve months', I smiled.

As I began my session, I reflected on how far I had come. That first day, when I walked into Anytime Fitness, my confidence was virtually non-existent. I was filled with embarrassment for how overweight I had become, and I had no idea what to do to improve my state. I wanted to achieve results, but I knew that it was not going to be done overnight. I allowed myself to enjoy the journey that I chose to be on, and the results came over time. A year later, I didn't need to worry about how I looked when I picked up a dumbbell or completed a set of walking lunges. Now, I was focused on myself and setting goals for my future, and the stress of how I looked had nearly faded.

When you get the opportunity to put yourself out there, it is normal to feel uncomfortable about doing it. You have two options: say yes to the opportunity and take yourself out of your comfort zone; or say no, only to look back further down the track wishing you had said yes. Of course, saying yes will expose you to things that are outside of your norm, but you need to trust the process. When you undergo this kind of transformation, allow yourself to look back and celebrate your achievements. Celebrate your milestones, especially the big ones, like a one-year anniversary. Although one year may feel like a short period, a lot can be achieved in this span of time, including taking steps into the unknown, making important sacrifices, and embarking on new opportunities. There is no better feeling than saying, 'I'm so glad I accomplished my goal!'

09

ANSWERING THE CALL TO ADVENTURE

Over the course of your transformation journey, you may have the opportunity to answer the call to adventure. In my case, this was an invitation to attend a life-changing self-development retreat. I want to encourage you to set out on the adventure, even if you have to make some sacrifices to get there. Saying 'yes' to the opportunity can lead to huge shifts in your personal growth. I'll tell you, when my opportunity came, I was hesitant at first as I did not know what to expect. As I later learned, I needed to trust the process and take that step into the unknown.

As I welcomed the new year, I felt like I was once again on the path of burn out. I didn't allow myself to take a break from my job, and I found myself working longer hours than I had the previous financial year. To be honest, I didn't even consider taking time off work. It was my manager, Lauren, who noticed that I was overdue for annual leave.

'Hey Oliver', Lauren asked me one morning, 'when was the last time you took leave, as in two weeks consecutively?'

I thought about it for a moment, and replied, 'It would have been more than a year ago.'

'When are you planning to take time off?' asked Lauren. 'I'm asking because you have a lot of annual leave accumulated.'

'I'm not sure', I said. 'I'll have to have a think about it. I'll let you know when I choose some annual leave dates.'

Later that evening whilst I was relaxing at home, I received a message from Charlotte, my life coach.

'Hi Oliver, hope you're keeping well. Just letting you know that I'm leading a retreat in Bali, and I've just had a cancellation. If this is something you'd like to do, there's a spot for you. Just have a think about it. I think you'd get a lot out of it.'

What a nice coincidence, I thought. A few days away was exactly what I was looking for. This could be perfect. I sent Charlotte a quick reply.

'Hi Charlotte, all is well for me. I really appreciate the offer, and I will definitely have a think about it.'

'Okay perfect. Get back to me as soon as you can. I am giving you first priority for the spot. I will send you a video promo of the program to help you decide. I think you will love it.'

A moment later, Charlotte sent me a link to the video. I saw tropical forest-like scenery at a private retreat. My immediate thought was that this setting would allow me to find peace. The description of the programme, including the service, meals, and meditation sessions made my decision easier.

'This looks incredible', I messaged Charlotte as soon as the video ended.

'I'm sure you will love it', Charlotte replied. 'Do what you need to do to arrange time off work and let me know how you go.'

'I will speak to my manager tomorrow', I typed. 'I'll let you know asap.'

'Perfect. I will keep the spot open for you', said Charlotte.

The next day, I submitted a request to take four days off in March.

'I'm sorry, Oliver. Unfortunately, we already have a few people taking time off during the days you have requested', said Lauren. 'Are there any other days you can take off?'

'I was hoping for these days specifically as I plan to be at a retreat in Bali', I said, shaking my head. I was flooded with feelings of disappointment as I made my way back home that evening.

I texted Charlotte as soon as I arrived home. 'I spoke to my manager today, and I couldn't get the time off I requested. It looks like I won't be able to go to Bali, after all.'

Charlotte's reply came later that evening. 'Oliver, I'm going to encourage you to speak to your manager tomorrow. This will be good practice for you in asking for what you want and making your needs clear. I think you will be able to work something out. I believe in you.'

'Okay. I'll definitely give it another try', I typed.

'Good! Let her know that you will only need the Thursday, Friday, and Monday off. The retreat is Thursday through Sunday. It's going to work out. I know it.'

I felt like my chances of going to the retreat were slipping through my fingers. I sensed the old, dark cloud of depression swirling around me. The next day, I wondered if I should just give up. After all, Lauren had told me that the week I had requested off wasn't available. Then, as I was about to take my lunch break, I got a text from Charlotte.

'Hi Oliver, have you had a chance to talk to your manager today?'

'Not yet', I replied.

'Don't give up hope. Ask her. You'll find a way.'

'Okay, I will.'

'Perfect. I'm still holding your spot in the retreat.'

I felt that my chances were slim, but I took on Charlotte's advice to try and work something out with my manager. 'Hey Lauren', I said as I approached her desk. 'I just wanted to touch base regarding my leave request. I was wondering if there's anything we can work out.'

'Unfortunately, there are three other people taking time off that week, as I mentioned. If you take a look here, there is no capacity for me to approve any more leave', said Lauren as she brought up the calendar on her computer.

I looked over her shoulder at her computer screen, and I instantly knew that Charlotte was right—there was a reason for me to double check. 'Oh, I actually was hoping to take the four days off in March. The calendar is showing April.'

Lauren's eyes widened, and she did a double take. 'Oh! I'm so sorry, Oliver. My mistake! I honestly don't know why I thought you requested for April.' She scrolled the calendar to March and looked at the dates I had requested. 'Those dates are available! I'll put in your leave request. That was very smart of you to triple check, just to make sure. Sorry about that! You're approved.'

I began to smile, mentally thanking Charlotte for encouraging me to persist. 'Thank you so much', I replied.

'Where in Bali are you staying?' asked Lauren.

'I will be in Ubud', I replied.

'Fantastic! Ubud is beautiful', she said. 'I'm so glad you'll be able to go!'

I sent Charlotte a message as soon as I finished work. 'I've just spoken to my manager, and she had unintentionally checked the wrong month before. We got everything straightened out, and I'm pleased to let you know that my leave has been approved, and I cannot wait to see you in Bali.'

"

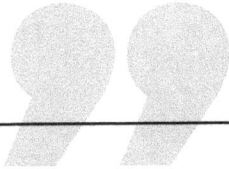

I WANT TO ENCOURAGE
YOU TO SET OUT ON THE
ADVENTURE, EVEN IF
YOU HAVE TO MAKE SOME
SACRIFICES TO GET THERE.
SAYING 'YES' TO THE
OPPORTUNITY CAN LEAD
TO HUGE SHIFTS IN YOUR
PERSONAL GROWTH.

A few hours later, I got a voicemail from Charlotte. 'How wonderful to hear your good news! I am glad you double checked. Good on you for advocating for yourself! Congratulations, and yes, the countdown to Bali begins.'

I wasted no time in paying the initial deposit for the retreat and booking my flights to Bali. The excitement only grew more as soon as I received my flight booking confirmation.

The next day, I had a coaching call with Charlotte, and the main topic was the upcoming retreat. 'I'm so glad that you double checked your leave request and got the green light', she said. 'I've been praying for a miracle, hoping that you will be able to attend.'

'Thank you so much for doing that', I replied.

'My pleasure. It just goes to show that prayers are powerful', she said.

'True. They really are', I smiled. 'This was also a good reminder that I need to advocate for myself more.'

'That's right!' said Charlotte. 'Be assertive, state your needs, and set boundaries. And most importantly, when you want something, never give up!'

> I THOUGHT TO MYSELF, 'I CAN'T BELIEVE I'M ACTUALLY HERE IN BALI. IF I HADN'T STUCK UP FOR MYSELF AT WORK, NONE OF THIS WOULD BE HAPPENING.' I FELT VERY PROUD THAT I HAD ADVOCATED FOR MYSELF. THIS WAS ONE OF THE CLEAREST EXAMPLES YET THAT MY EXPERIENCES WERE A DIRECT RESULT OF MY CHOICES AND ACTIONS.

The months flew by, and soon the day came for me to leave for Bali. I made my way to the airport and went through check-in and security with relative ease. As I arrived at my gate, I saw a Jetstar Dreamliner parked outside. This was the magnificent airplane that would take me to Denpasar, Bali's capital city. It wasn't long until we began to board the flight, and I found my seat in the rear section of the aircraft, behind the engines. We pushed back on schedule and took off towards the west for a five-hour flight. I passed the time listening to music and watching a few episodes of *The Big Bang Theory*, and soon we began our descent towards Bali, landing nearly half an hour ahead of schedule. There was a slight culture shock when I cleared customs and made my way out into the arrival hall. As I looked around me to get my bearings, I saw a driver holding up my name and flight number.

'Hi, I'm Oliver', I said to the driver, letting out a sigh of relief.

'Hi, please come with me', said the driver as he took my suitcase and led me out towards the car. 'Welcome to Denpasar.'

'Thank you, it's great to be back', I replied.

'When was the last time you were in Bali?' asked the driver as we left the airport carpark.

'More than twenty years ago', I replied. 'I came here when I was eight.'

'That is a long time to be away', said the driver. 'Welcome back.'

An hour later, the driver pulled into a little back street. 'Okay, we are here. We'll need to walk down that path', he said, pointing to a winding dirt road. 'The villa is that way.'

I nodded, and we made our way along the gravelly path. Soon, I heard people's voices.

'Your guest has arrived', announced the driver as we entered the villa.

I looked over and saw Charlotte standing in front of a bungalow-style house with a thatched roof. There were many such buildings that lined the little dirt road. She was surrounded by a group of other guests.

'Hey Oliver!' called Charlotte. 'Come meet everybody! This is Layla, John, Jean, and Melenaite.'

'Please, just call me Mel', said a woman standing beside Charlotte. 'It's so nice to meet you, Oliver. I've been following your journey on Instagram.'

'I'm Jean. Good to meet you. Mel and I are working with Charlotte too.'

'Yes, it's nice to meet you, Oliver. I'm Layla. I'm tag-teaming Charlotte as coach. This is sort of a working vacation for me. I'm a nutritionist, so I'm doing the meal planning for all of us.'

'It's great to meet all of you', I said. 'I'm really excited to be here.'

'How long was the flight up to Bali?' asked John.

'It was just about five hours', I replied.

'That's not bad, compared to a twenty-hour flight from Dallas', laughed John. 'Charlotte and I met at a retreat in Texas a few years back. I'm here as her videographer. You've been one of her clients for a little while, right?'

'Yeah, I've worked with her over the past three years' I said. 'This last year has been incredible. I've lost nearly 30kg.'

'Wow! Do the conversion for me', said John. 'How much is that in pounds?'

'It's over 60lbs', I said.

'Good for you!' nodded John. 'Here, let me show you something.' He reached into his pocket to pull out his phone. 'This was my weight loss transformation from a number of years ago', he said, showing me a before--and-after picture.

'That's a huge difference!' I said, looking at his phone screen. His health journey was evident in the side-by-side photos.

'Thanks. It was a lot of hard work to get from A to B', said John.

'I don't doubt you for a minute', I said. 'Thanks for showing me your transformation. It's really motivating for me to see other people going through the same thing.'

'I think we should have our main meal now', said Charlotte. 'All activities and meals will be held in our bungalow.' She nodded to the large, hut-like building behind her. 'Oliver, your bedroom is down the hall and to the right. There's also a pool out back for you all to enjoy. Today, let's get to bed early. We have a full day ahead of us tomorrow.'

After a restful night's sleep, I woke early in the morning and looked out the front door of our rented bungalow to witness the first oranges and pinks of the sunrise stretching across the sky. I got changed and sat outside by the pool.

'Morning Oliver, how did you sleep last night?' asked Mel as she walked out to join me.

'Morning, Mel. I slept quite well actually', I replied. 'I fell straight asleep as soon as I lay down.'

'Same, I was exhausted after yesterday', said Mel.

'So was I. I was awake since 4:00 a.m. Melbourne time yesterday. At least I don't feel too jetlagged today.'

It wasn't long until the rest of the guests were awake, and we made our way to the dining area for breakfast. I opted in for coconut pancakes with honey, berries, and melon. The fruit practically melted in my mouth as I ate it, it was so fresh.

'As soon as we finish breakfast, we will head to a spa in Ubud', announced Charlotte.

Jean looked up from a journal she was writing in. 'I can't wait to get a massage. It's been too long!'

A half hour later, Charlotte called for our transportation, and we were on our way to the best rated spa in Ubud.

When we arrived at the spa, we met with the concierge, who gave us each an intake form and a menu of treatment options to choose from. 'I think I'm getting a 90-minute massage and a detox bath', I said as I looked at the paperwork.

'That actually sounds really good', said Layla. 'Where's the detox bath listed?'

'It's right here', I said, pointing to the menu.

'Thanks, Oliver', said Layla, completing her form.

I smiled. It felt nice to be able to help someone out. After a short wait, we got called to our respective rooms. I followed an attendant down a flight of stairs and along a narrow hallway to a private treatment chamber with a massage table and a bath. The sunlit room was framed on three sides by large, screened-in windows, allowing the sounds and smells of nature to permeate the space.

'I will give you time to undress. Once you are ready, please lie face down on the massage table', said the masseuse.

'Where should I leave my clothes?' I asked.

'There is a coat hanger you can place your clothes on', replied the masseuse as she made her way out of the room.

I got ready within five minutes and climbed face-down onto the massage table, pulling a thin, white sheet over my back. A little while later, the masseuse returned and began my massage. Within a few minutes, I felt the tension from the last few days starting to melt away. My whole being was flooded with feelings of relaxation and calm.

As I lay there, I thought to myself, 'I can't believe I'm actually here in Bali. If I hadn't stuck up for myself at work, none of this would be happening.' I felt very proud that I had advocated for myself. This was one of the clearest examples yet that my experiences were a direct result of my choices and actions.

As my massage drew to a close, another spa attendant came into the room to prepare the detox portion of my treatment. I could hear the gentle sound of flowing water as a lightly sulphurous aroma filled my nostrils, mixed with the scent of essential oils.

'The bath is ready for you now', said the masseuse. 'It contains magnesium sulphate and other detoxification agents. I will leave you now and give you time to transition. We have also provided you with citrus water and a plate of high alkaline fruits for you to enjoy.'

'Okay, thank you', I murmured, still in a state of deep relaxation. After the masseuse left, I slowly climbed off the table and stepped into the bath. The water was warm, nearly hot. It took me a minute to lower my body into the bathtub without overheating. To my right was a little table with a jug of citrus water, a cut crystal glass, and a plate filled with melons, dragon fruit, and pineapple. I helped myself to a full glass of the water, which was surprisingly refreshing. Then I sank back into the bath and nibbled on the fruit. Within minutes, sweat started pouring down my brow. I figured this must be a result of the detox agents in the water.

I'M GOING TO CHALLENGE YOU A LITTLE BIT. IT MAY BE THE CASE THAT YOU ARE GENUINELY SATISFIED AT WORK, BUT I WANT YOU TO HAVE A DEEPER THINK ABOUT IT. WHAT DO YOU WANT TO DO AS A CAREER? I THINK YOU MAY BE FOCUSSING TOO MUCH ON WHAT YOU ARE DOING AND NOT THINKING ABOUT WHAT YOU ACTUALLY WANT TO DO.'

Too soon, an attendant knocked on the door. 'You have twenty more minutes for your detox, and then you will have five minutes to dress.'

'Okay, thank you', I called out through a mouthful of melon.

As the 30-minute bath came to an end, I dried myself off and changed back into my clothes. I began sweating profusely as I walked up the stairs to the main spa entrance. Charlotte and Mel were already there.

'How amazing was that?' asked Mel.

'I loved it, but I can't stop sweating from the detox bath', I laughed.

'It looks as though your body is still flushing out the toxins', said Charlotte. 'That's good!'

Soon, the rest of the retreat group returned to the main entrance, and we made our way back to the villa for dinner and our group coaching session. Today, Charlotte was coaching us on designing our ideal environment.

'I'd like you to describe your perfect day, your perfect job, and how you picture it all going', she said. 'We'll go one-by-one around the room.'

When it was my turn, I said, 'I think my perfect day would be coming into work, doing my usual routine at my job, and then going to the gym to train. I don't know what my perfect job would be, so I'm not sure if I can answer that part of the question.'

Charlotte looked at me with an odd expression on her face. 'Really?' she said. 'Is that really your ideal day at your ideal job? Now, Oliver, I'm going to challenge you a little bit. It may be the case that you are genuinely satisfied at work, but I want you to have a deeper think about it. What do you want to do as a career? I think you may be focussing too much on what you are doing and not thinking about what you actually want to do.'

I was silent for a moment as I tried to process Charlotte's words. 'I guess I haven't ever considered whether I'm happy at work. I know that my job is sometimes draining, but I've never really thought about doing anything else. As for a career, I genuinely have no idea what I would want to do. I'll have to have a think about it.'

'I hope this exercise will help you gain more clarity on what you really want out of your life and work, Oliver. You've got a lot to offer this world.'

Little did I know how much this simple coaching exercise would soon help me expand my outlook on life.

If you receive an invitation to attend a transforma-
tional event, like a seminar or a retreat, chances
are that this has happened for a reason. It may
be daunting at first, but it will open up opportunities that you hadn't even considered. You will
meet others who will be inspired by the path you
are on. They will want to hear your story and learn
from the hardships and sacrifices you have gone
through. You will do yourself a favour if you say 'yes'
and commit to the journey.

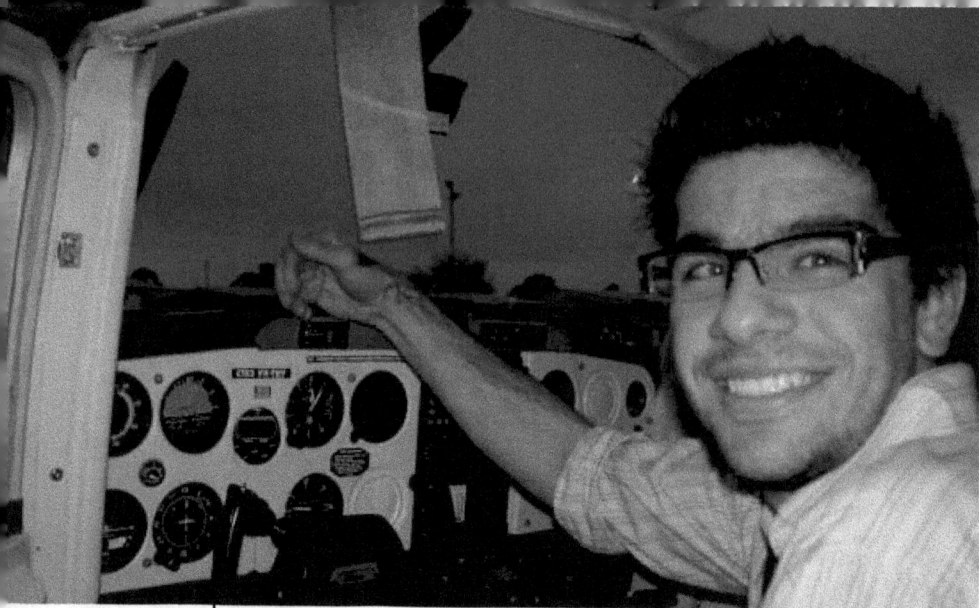

Flight training — This was after I arrived from one of my solo sessions, completing circuits around Tyabb Airfield. Photographer — David Bell

Gratitude and forgiveness in Bali — This was during our group session at the Bali retreat. I had just written down the list of what I forgave, and I was experiencing a breakthrough. Charlotte offered burnt sage as I was completing my heart-focussed breathing. Photographer — Jonathan Taylor

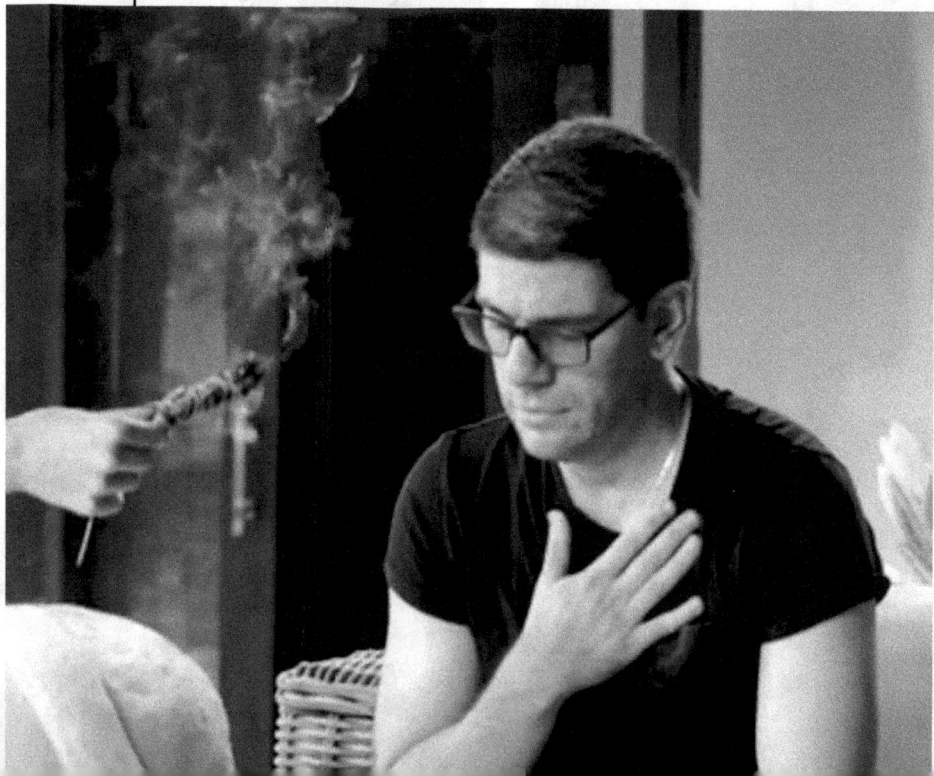

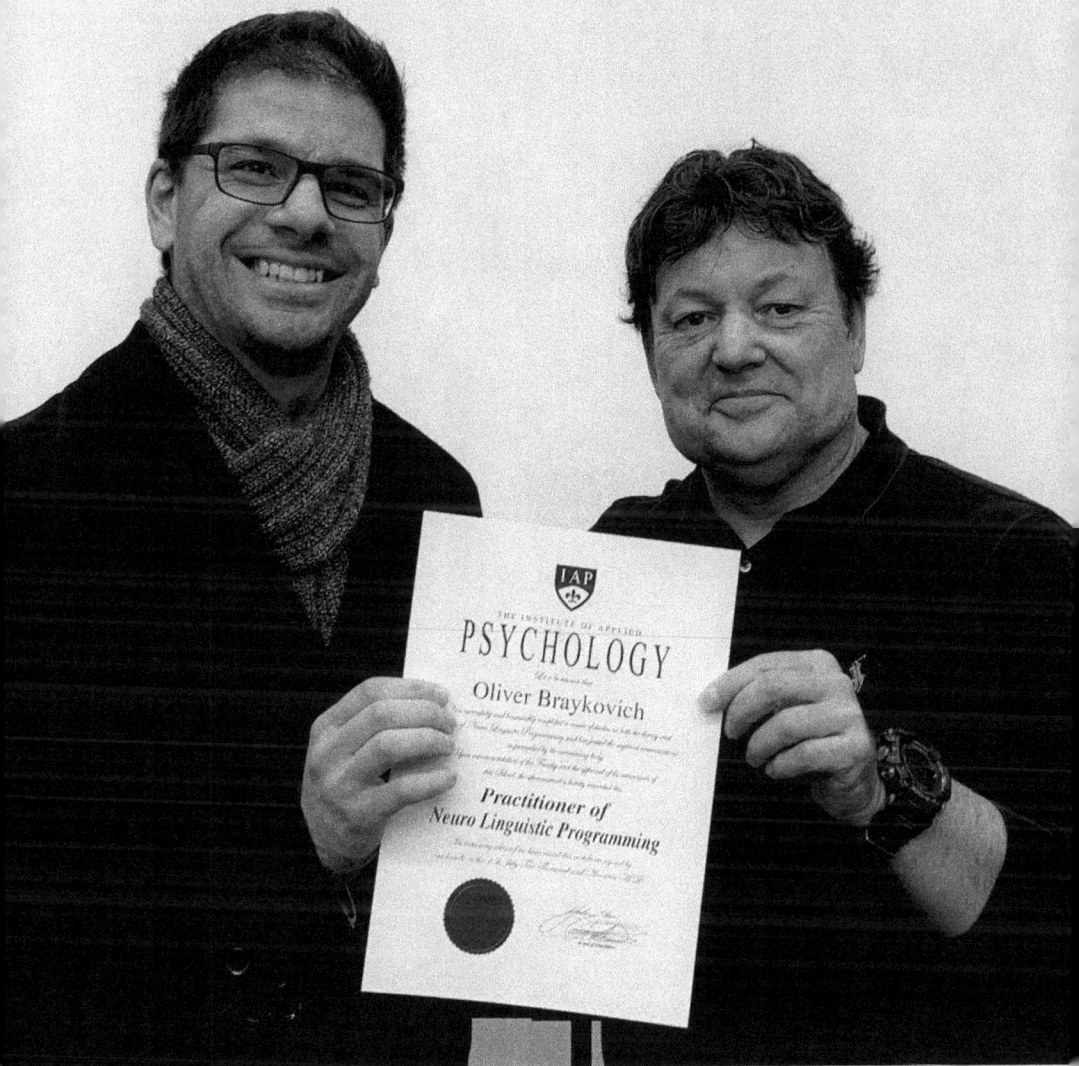

Receiving my NLP certificate from Gordon Young — This was upon my completion of the NLP Practitioner course, where I received my certificate after achieving 100% in the module's final assessment. Photographer — Unknown

LETTING GO

One of the biggest steps you will take along your journey is learning how to let go. This may be forgiving past relationships or releasing negative emotions that you have been bottling up for years. Once you do, your growth and confidence will improve, and you may find that new opportunities will appear unexpectedly. It won't be easy, but allowing yourself to experience gratitude and forgiveness will lift a huge weight off your shoulders and set you on a path of healing.

The next morning, I awoke and went straight to morning meditation and then ate a delicious breakfast of fruit and pancakes. After breakfast, we gathered in the group coaching room, and Charlotte announced our next session.

'Today, we will be focussing on gratitude and forgiveness', she said, taking out a bundle of sage. 'This is not about forgiving others; instead, you will be learning to forgive yourselves. This is a powerful practice, and you will feel a lot of emotions arise as you are going through the process. It will prepare you for the water ceremony this evening, where you will be able to fully let go of what is holding you back.'

I wasn't sure how to feel at the time. I didn't know if I was even ready to go through this process, but I knew I had to take this step if I wanted to move forward in my life.

'I want you all to take out your journals and write down everything that you forgive yourself for', Charlotte continued. 'Then I want you to write down all the ways you celebrate yourself.' She lit the sage and began smudging the room. 'This is a free association exercise. You don't have to come up with any structure. Just write down whatever comes to mind.'

Charlotte turned on some peaceful music to help set the mood. I took out my journal and began writing.

I forgive myself for spiralling into anxiety and depression. I forgive myself for not looking after my health. I forgive myself for feeling sorry for myself. I forgive myself for always holding back and letting my fear get in my way. I forgive myself for not standing up for myself. I forgive myself for being angry with other people for no reason. I forgive myself for being so afraid all the time.

As I wrote, I began to tremble. Tears brimmed in my eyes and threatened to spill down my cheeks. I wiped at my eyes to hide the evidence of my emotions. As I looked around, I saw Charlotte walking towards Mel, holding out a box of tissues. Tears were streaming down Mel's face as she quietly sobbed.

'Charlotte?' I asked as she returned to the middle of the room. 'I'm shaking. Is that normal?'

'Yes, it can be', Charlotte responded. 'Place your hand on your chest and focus your breathing on your heart.'

She picked up the sage again and began another round of smudging. I closed my eyes and began breathing into my heart centre, allowing the scent of the sage to calm me. In that moment, all the negative emotions that I had supressed for the past fourteen years began to rise to the surface. I began to cry. I forgave myself for the deep cloud of depression that had hung over my head throughout my childhood. I forgave myself for all the difficulties I'd had in connecting with people. I forgave myself for not knowing how to stick up for myself or set clear boundaries.

I had a sense of clarity that I was ready to let go and begin moving forward with my life. I also felt like I was finally able to acknowledge and celebrate all the things I had accomplished along my journey. I continued writing in my journal.

I celebrate myself for transforming my life. I celebrate myself for going to the gym six days a week. I celebrate myself for being alive every day. I celebrate myself for stepping out of my comfort zone. I celebrate myself for saying yes to every opportunity that comes to me. I celebrate myself for committing to my meal planning. I celebrate myself for being the amazing person that I am today.

At that moment, I realised that I deserved self-forgiveness. I gave myself permission to let go of the blame, guilt, and shame I had carried for so long.

The rest of the afternoon passed in a blur. That evening, we all climbed in a van that would take us to the Tirta Empu temple for the water ceremony. When we arrived, we went to a changing room to put on swimwear as we would be entering the sacred pool. Then Charlotte gave us each a piece of ceremonial temple clothing to drape over our shoulders.

> **I REALISED THAT I DESERVED SELF-FORGIVENESS. I GAVE MYSELF PERMISSION TO LET GO OF THE BLAME, GUILT, AND SHAME I HAD CARRIED FOR SO LONG.**

'As you walk into the pool, you will see many different fountains', said Charlotte. 'I will show you which ones we will be using.'

As I approached the pool, I was amazed to see how beautiful the fountains were. They glistened and danced in the flickering light cast by flaming torches that lined the temple walls.

'You will be using these twelve fountains', said Charlotte, gesturing towards several fountains in front of us. 'As you approach each one, you will splash water over your head three times, over your face three times, and then dunk your head under the fountain.'

I was the first to lower myself into the water and take that next important step of letting go.

'Wait, don't go any further', said John, pointing to the other side of the pool. 'There's a snake over there.'

I froze.

'Is it venomous?' asked Jean.

'I hope not', I said. 'I'm going to stay really still.'

'It's okay!' said Charlotte. 'I forgot to mention it. The staff warned me that we might see them, but they assured me that they're not venomous.'

I nodded and waded further into the pool, catching my breath as the chilly water swirled around my waist. I went straight to the first fountain, and I didn't flinch, even when the snake slithered along the edge of the pool. 'It's okay', I whispered to myself. 'It can't hurt me. After all, a snake is a symbol of rebirth.' As I stood in front of the fountain, I followed Charlotte's instructions. I splashed the water over my head three times, again over my face three times, and then I placed my head under the running fountain. I looked back at Charlotte, and she gave me a thumbs up. I nodded and made my way to the second fountain.

As I repeated the same process at the rest of the twelve fountains,

I felt the burdensome emotions I'd been carrying rise to the surface and then slip away into the purifying water. Finally, I reached the last fountain. I repeated the same ritual, this time placing my head under the cascading water for more than thirty seconds, allowing it to wash away the last of the negative emotions I'd been harbouring for the past fourteen years.

'How was it, Oliver?' asked Charlotte as she helped me out of the pool. I struggled to find the words. An indescribable emotion welled within me. I felt like I might burst into tears, or maybe laughter. 'I didn't realise how powerful this process is. Thank you, Charlotte.' I reached out to give her a hug. Eyes closed, we held onto each other for a wordless minute. 'I've finally been able to let go', I said.

'You did so well, and I am so proud of you', she whispered into my ear. 'This will be an experience you will never forget.'

As Layla, Jean, and Mel waded out of the pool, we all sat by the edge to wait for John to emerge. Finally, Charlotte stepped into the water to take her turn. Fifteen minutes later, she returned to the group, a broad grin illuminating her face.

'That really was magical', she said. 'I'm so grateful that I got to share this experience with all of you.'

We travelled back to the villa in silence, each of us processing the transformation we had just undergone. With sleep-filled eyes, I climbed out of the van and walked slowly to the kitchen, where I made myself a cup of herbal tea. Feeling exhausted, I said goodnight to the rest of the guests and stumbled my way to my room, where I fell into a deep sleep, filled with dreams of snakes shedding their skin.

The next morning, I awoke at 6:00 a.m., feeling refreshed and energized after the exhausting previous day. As I walked outside to watch the sunrise, I saw Jean emerge from the bungalow to greet the dawn.

'Morning, Oliver. Did you sleep well?' she asked, gazing at the sky.

'Morning, Jean', I said. 'I slept like a rock last night. I was exhausted after the water ceremony.'

'Yeah, I know. That ceremony knocked me right out', said Jean.

'Not that I'm complaining', I smiled. 'I had a major breakthrough. I let go of so much baggage, I feel like I'm ten pounds lighter.'

Jean and I chuckled at my joke. We made our way to the dining room and began our breakfast. Slowly, the other guests arrived as well.

'Morning all', said Charlotte as she emerged from her room. 'We have another big day ahead of us. Today is the fire ceremony. Before that, we'll have our one-on-one sessions. Oliver, I'd like to ask you to go first this morning.'

'Okay', I nodded. An hour later, I went to see Charlotte for my private session. I sat quietly in the private coaching room, allowing the calming smell of sage to wash over me.

'So, Oliver', said Charlotte. 'Today, I'd like to revisit the exercise where you imagine your ideal day and your ideal job. Could you tell me more about your ideal day?'

I thought for a moment. 'Well, I guess my ideal day is to go to work, train at the gym, and spend time with my ideal partner.'

'Okay, that's a good start', said Charlotte. 'Would going to your current job be part of your ideal day? Or do you imagine a different career path, like helping others?'

'I'm honestly not too sure about my current work being part of my ideal day', I replied, shaking my head.

'It's perfectly okay if it is', said Charlotte. 'If you're happy where you are, that's great.'

'I do want to help others, though', I said. 'I guess, if I altered my ideal day, I would change the work I do from my current job to, say, being a personal trainer.'

'Okay! I would like to do a heart-focussed breathing session around that change', said Charlotte. 'You can lie down for this if you want to.' She gestured to a large couch in the middle of the room.

I nodded and lay down across the couch cushions. The smell of sage wafted all around me, growing stronger with each breath.

'Now, close your eyes', said Charlotte. 'Breathe in and breathe out. Imagine breathing into your heart. Open yourself up to the gratitude you feel for yourself, for this space, for the people around you. Feel the gratitude for the path you are travelling—where you were, where you are, and where you will be.'

'I think I know what I need to do', I said quietly. 'I definitely need to rethink my ideal day and put my plans into action.'

I opened my eyes and slowly stood up. Charlotte opened her arms to give me a hug.

'Remember, Oliver, you are living proof that you can do anything that you set your mind to.'

'It's definitely not impossible', I nodded.

'That's right. It's doable. It might be difficult, but remember Oliver, you can do difficult things', said Charlotte, looking in my eyes. 'Since the beginning of last year, you have been walking your talk, and you are just smashing your goals left, right, and centre.'

I left my coaching session with a lot to think about. Opportunities were starting to appear on the horizon. I just needed to stay open to possibility.

It was not long before we were called to prepare for the fire ceremony. Charlotte had arranged for another SUV to take us to a place about a half hour from the villa. She led us along a forest path to a clearing, where a large fire roared within a circular firepit. As we approached, we were greeted by a High Priest in ceremonial robes, who gave us each a pair of small, wooden bowls. I thanked him and looked down to examine the contents. In one bowl, there was an assortment of various seeds. In the other, there was a whole coconut. I raised my eyebrows. I wondered if I was supposed to eat these.

Once we all had received our bowls, the High Priest spoke, answering my unstated question. 'When I say "swaha", you throw the seeds into the fire. Then you repeat the prayer, "swaha". Throw the seeds and repeat the prayer until you have only one handful left. Don't throw this final handful just yet.'

The High Priest started chanting a prayer in a language I didn't understand. Then, I heard the word I was listening for. 'Swaha!'

I took a handful of seeds and tossed them into the fire. 'Swaha!' I yelled. I grabbed another handful and threw it. 'Swaha!' The seeds caused the fire to flutter and spark. I took one more handful, leaving a few seeds at the bottom of the bowl, and I cast it into the circle of flames. 'Swaha!'

'Good! This will bring you the success you wish for', said the High Priest. 'Now that you have thrown the seeds, take the bowl with the coconut. Smash the coconut onto the sharp rock over there.' He pointed to a jagged rock formation a few metres from the firepit. 'Once the coconut breaks in half, let the water inside flow from it onto the ground. Then, bring your coconut back to the circle and cast it into the fire.'

The six of us walked over to the jagged rock and began hitting our coconuts onto the sharp, stony surface. In the light of the fire, I saw that the rock was covered in dark stains. I wondered how many generations had participated in this ceremony before me. I smashed my coconut over and over until suddenly it split in half. Shards flew off onto the ground, and the water in the coconut poured through my fingers, staining the ceremonial rock with a fresh layer of patina. I picked up the pieces of my coconut and walked back to the fire. I threw it bit by bit into the flames until all that was left was the slight residue of the coconut water on my hands.

> I NODDED AND WADED FURTHER INTO THE POOL, CATCHING MY BREATH AS THE CHILLY WATER SWIRLED AROUND MY WAIST. I WENT STRAIGHT TO THE FIRST FOUNTAIN, AND I DIDN'T FLINCH, EVEN WHEN THE SNAKE SLITHERED ALONG THE EDGE OF THE POOL. 'IT'S OKAY', I WHISPERED TO MYSELF. 'IT CAN'T HURT ME. AFTER ALL, A SNAKE IS A SYMBOL OF REBIRTH.'

'Good!' said the High Priest. 'This will bring you happiness, money, and success for the future. Now, I want each of you to approach me. I will give you your next gift.'

As I walked up to the priest, he grabbed my right arm. He reached into a bag and took out three thin wristbands—one black, one red, and one white. He slid them one by one onto my wrist, saying, 'Black is for wealth and for the feeling of groundedness that comes from the earth. Red is for protection from past hurts. White is for pure, unconditional love.' Then, he let go of my arm and motioned for me to return.

'Take your bowls', he instructed once we all had our wristbands. 'Throw your last handful of seeds onto the fire. Once you do, the ceremony will be complete.'

We gathered the rest of our seeds and threw them into the fire. As we did, the High Priest came round the circle to hug each of us. 'Thank you for coming', he said. 'I wish you all the success for the future.'

We soon left and returned to the villa for our farewell dinner. I was silent for most of the meal, processing the ritual I had just experienced. As we were finishing our dessert, Charlotte told us, 'Come over by the pool area when you're done. I have a surprise for you all.'

We made our way outside, and Charlotte opened a box filled with paper lanterns, one for each of us. 'I will hand you a lantern to unfold', she said. 'As I do, I will light a candle inside. The heat from the candle will cause the lantern to rise. Hold onto your lantern until you feel the upward pull. Once you feel this pull, think of something that you are ready to let go of. When the time is right, let go of the lantern, and as you do, let go of the thing that you have been holding onto.'

I took my lantern and unfolded it, expanding it into its circular shape. Charlotte lit a tall wax candle and placed it inside. I held onto the delicate paper, waiting for the upward pressure to build. I already knew what I was ready to let go of. I whispered to myself, 'I am ready to let go of my fear of connecting with people. I will no longer be scared of what others think of me.'

At that moment, I let go of the lantern. Slowly, it rose from my hands and drifted upwards, carried away by the gentle evening breeze. As I watched it float into the sky, I allowed it to carry away the social anxieties and fears that I had swaddled myself with for so long. I looked around at the group. Layla was standing with her hands pressed against her heart. Mel was wiping away tears that flowed in little rivulets down her cheeks. Jean was staring at her lantern, a hopeful expression lighting her face.

'Come on, everyone', said Charlotte. 'Let's have a group hug.'

We hugged and cried, celebrating our newfound bond. We were not the same people we had been just a few days before. We had all been shaped by the profound experience of personal transformation.

It is normal to carry negative emotions, whether it is from past relationships or bad experiences in school. You will make it difficult for yourself to grow if you hold onto these emotions. Forgiveness is the key to letting go and releasing this burden. Forgive others, and most importantly, forgive yourself. This may be a difficult step, but as you begin your forgiveness journey, a weight will begin to lift off your shoulders. As you go through the process of forgiving yourself, remember it is just as important to show yourself and others around you your gratitude. Celebrate yourself. You deserve it.

FINDING MY PURPOSE

It is often difficult to find your true passion; in fact, it may take you years to find something that you are destined for. As soon as you come to the realization that 'this is my calling in life', you will want to reach out to a coach who can help you turn that desire into a reality. I struggled for many years to find what it was that I really wanted to do. This led to frustration and burn out. Finally, I found my true calling. My purpose is to be a beacon of light to help others through the same dark path that I travelled.

Soon it was time for me to return home from Bali. I flew back to Melbourne the next day, and by Wednesday morning, I was once again at my desk. As I finished work for the day, I made my way to Anytime Fitness for my training session.

'Hey, Oli! how was your trip?' asked William as I started my warmup.

'It was incredible', I said. 'I'll never forget it.'

'That is awesome to hear', said William. 'You look good. You seem more centred than you did before.'

'I've gone through such a huge transformation, Will', I said. 'Honestly, this retreat has changed my life.'

'Wow, I can see that it's had a huge impact on you!'

'I had some amazing coaching sessions there, both group coaching and one-on-one. Actually, I wanted to run something by you', I said, taking a deep breath. 'Whilst I was there, I had a realization. It almost felt like a calling. I'm wondering what it would be like to become a life coach.'

'Man, you would be a great mentor', said William. 'I'd say, go for it! Your story has inspired so many people already. There are a lot of people that you could help as a coach. Think of all the guys who are where you were a year and a half ago. They're fed up with being fed up, but they don't know what to do to make things better. You could help those people, Oli. You could show them how to change their life.'

As I sat on the train home that evening, I played William's words over in my mind. The more I thought about it, the clearer I became that my life's purpose is to help others overcome depression and learn to win at life. I knew at that point that I had to take action and look for a programme that would help me achieve my goal.

In the coming days, I started searching for life coaching courses. As I thought about my coaching prospects even more, the Institute of Applied Psychology in Sydney stood out to me. Finally, I gathered my courage, and I submitted my query to the Institute.

The next morning, I received a phone call from Brigitte, a career advisor at the Institute.

'I understand that you want to apply for our coaching course', she said. 'I just want to clarify as to why you are interested in studying this course with us?'

'Well, this might sound a bit dramatic', I admitted, taking a deep breath, 'but I recently found my purpose. I was on a retreat in Bali, and I realised that my purpose is to become a coach. I've gone through coaching as a client for several years, so I know what it's like. I know how powerful and transformative it can be.'

'Going through coaching as a client is invaluable when it comes to coaching qualifications', said Brigitte. 'We do have a coaching program where you obtain your NLP strategic coaching and master practitioner certifications, as well as a facilitator qualification.'

'I'm definitely interested in going for the full course, all the way to facilitator', I replied.

'Fantastic. Just so you know, most of our classes will be in Sydney', said Brigitte. 'So, if you are from interstate, we will arrange $1,000 worth of travel vouchers, which we'll deduct from our total cost of the course.'

'That actually sounds amazing. I am more than happy to commit to travelling interstate to attend the classes', I replied. 'I'm so excited to begin my training!'

Soon, the first day of my NLP Leadership and Coaching course had arrived. It was a multi-weekend course, and if we passed it, we would be awarded an NLP certificate that would allow us to start our own life coaching practice. I made my way to Abbotsford Convent, where the training was being held. I had learnt from the welcome packet for the course that Master Practitioner Gordon Young would be my instructor. I still couldn't believe my luck. He was an internationally renowned trainer, and I was thrilled that I would be learning from the best.

I walked through the classroom door and saw Gordon Young standing in front of a room filled with other trainees.

'Good afternoon', he said as I looked around the room for an empty seat. 'I take it you are here for the practitioner course.'

'Yes, I am', I said, reminding myself to be assertive. I walked up to Gordon and extended my hand. 'I'm Oliver. Pleasure to meet you.'

'The pleasure is mine, Oliver. Please, find a seat. We'll get started soon.'

More students arrived in the room before class began. A man walked over to my table and sat in the seat beside me. He smiled and extended his hand.

'I'm Justin. Good to meet you. How're you going?'

'Going great. I'm Oliver, by the way', I said, shaking his hand. 'I'm finally taking action to achieve my purpose.'

'Good onya! That's really awesome to hear', said Justin. 'I'm here to learn NLP. It'll help me expand my coaching practice.'

'Okay, let's get started!' said Gordon, clapping his hands together to get everybody's attention. 'Welcome everyone. For those who don't know me, I'm Gordon Young. I am the founder of The Institute of Applied Psychology. I'm a registered Clinical Hypnotherapist and an NLP Master Practitioner. In this class, I will be pushing you to your limits. You will often feel overwhelmed and irritated. That's to be expected. It's designed to help you make the breakthroughs you need in order to become a coach.'

That day, we spent time completing a Wheel of Life assessment to seek out imbalances in our life.

There were ten key areas that the test highlighted:

> I THOUGHT BACK TO ONLY A FEW YEARS AGO. MY WHEEL OF LIFE HAD BEEN SO IMBALANCED BACK THEN. I SMILED, THINKING ABOUT HOW MUCH I HAD GROWN IN A SHORT AMOUNT OF TIME.

- Family
- Friends
- Health
- Career
- Money
- Relationships
- Fun
- Higher Purpose
- Personal Development
- Physical Environment

We were to rate ourselves on a scale of 1–10 in each area, a score of 10 being the highest. I was not surprised to find that I scored the lowest on Relationships. I knew I still needed to work on that area of my life. Still, I was pleased to see that I scored myself highly in many other areas, especially Health, Friends, Family, and Personal Development. I thought back to only a few years ago. My Wheel of Life had been so imbalanced back then. I smiled, thinking about how much I had grown in a short amount of time.

The next day, Gordon announced, 'We are now going to move onto Belief Change. This exercise will tackle the critical inner voice, and it will show you how to do a pattern interrupt on yourself and others. Now, I'm not going to ask for a volunteer. I am going to feel out who needs a change of beliefs.' Gordon walked over to where I was sitting. 'There is someone in this area who has a specific fear-based belief, and I want to address it.'

Gordon waved his hand in my direction. In that moment, I knew that somehow, he could sense the fear that constantly cycled around in the back of my mind. Before I could stop myself, I blurted out, 'I can never be loved!'

'There it is. There's the limiting belief', said Gordon as he pointed towards me. 'Come on up to the front of the class.'

I felt like I was about to cry. 'How did you know that I was thinking that?' I asked.

'I felt a strong indication that this was your belief. If I have your permission, I would like to tackle it.'

I swallowed hard. Then I nodded.

'Now, what comes to mind when you say that you can never be loved?' asked Gordon.

'Loneliness is what comes to mind first. That, and thinking that others don't really care about me', I said, my voice barely above a whisper.

'Okay, let's explore that a little more and work on it', said Gordon. 'I want you to tell me some things that you know to be true in your life. Tell me a fact about yourself that was true in your childhood but isn't true now. Then tell me a fact about yourself that is true today.'

'Well, a fact about me that was previously true is that I used to be able to play the violin', I said. 'I played when I was a child, but I can't play now.'

'And a fact about you that is true now?' asked Gordon. 'Don't overthink it. Just whatever comes to mind first.'

'Something true now is that I live in a double-storey home.'

'Great. These are two facts that you know to be true. One was true earlier in your life, and one is true now. So, how do you feel about the statement you made before? Could you repeat it?' asked Gordon.

I bowed my head. 'What I said before was, "I can never be loved".'

'And based on this exercise, would you now say with complete assuredness that this is a fact?' asked Gordon.

'No, I don't think it's a fact, actually', I said.

'Would you say that it is a belief, but not a fact?' asked Gordon.

'Yeah, I think so', I said.

'And would you say that it is a belief that limits you?' Gordon pressed.

'Yeah, that's a fair assessment', I replied.

'So, what would you say that you get out of this limiting belief?' asked Gordon. 'What's the payoff? What's the emotional reward?'

'Well, I guess that when I tell myself that limiting belief, it lets me off the hook', I whispered. 'I can just say to myself, "I can never be loved". Then I don't have to put myself out there. I can avoid rejection.' I felt tears welling in my eyes.

'That's a big realisation, Oliver', said Gordon gently. 'I want you to let yourself really feel that. You can absolutely be loved. You deserve to be loved. And there are people out there who will love you. Your job is to overcome the *fear* of being loved. Because right now, your brain associates love with rejection. Today, right now, you get to form a new association. Love is no longer about rejection. Now and forevermore, when you think about love, you will associate it with connection. So, Oliver, how do you feel now?'

I began to tremble. 'I feel that I can be loved. Love is about connection. I deserve love. I am loveable.'

'Good!' said Gordon, clapping his hands together. 'Now, what are your immediate thoughts when I tell you, "Oliver, you can never be loved"?'

'Well, that's your opinion', I replied.

'Yes! Good!' exclaimed Gordon.

'I do deserve love!' I said, my voice rising to a shout. 'And I am well and truly deserving of it, just like everyone else!'

Gordon beamed and started applauding. Soon, the rest of the class was cheering me on.

'I think I just had a breakthrough', I said.

After the class was over, I leapt up from my seat and rushed over to Gordon.

'I just want to say thank you for what you have done', I said as I shook Gordon's hand.

'It is my absolute pleasure', replied Gordon, 'but you're the one who did it.'

'Onwards and upwards', I smiled.

'That's it', nodded Gordon, clapping me on the shoulder. 'Onwards and upwards.'

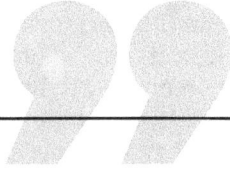

YOU CAN ABSOLUTELY BE LOVED. YOU DESERVE TO BE LOVED. AND THERE ARE PEOPLE OUT THERE WHO WILL LOVE YOU. YOUR JOB IS TO OVERCOME THE FEAR OF BEING LOVED. BECAUSE RIGHT NOW, YOUR BRAIN ASSOCIATES LOVE WITH REJECTION. TODAY, RIGHT NOW, YOU GET TO FORM A NEW ASSOCIATION. LOVE IS NO LONGER ABOUT REJECTION. NOW AND FOREVERMORE, WHEN YOU THINK ABOUT LOVE, YOU WILL ASSOCIATE IT WITH CONNECTION.

The following weekend, I began reviewing the NLP coursebook to prepare for my assessment. If I passed, I would receive a strategic coaching certification, and I would be on my way to becoming an NLP master practitioner. I made sure to study every module in enough depth that I could commit the coursebook to memory. I was determined to get a good grade. I woke up early on the day of the test and finished the assessment in an hour and a half. When I answered the final problem, the testing program informed me that my instructor would tell me whether I had passed. I sighed. I would have liked to have seen my score there and then, but I knew I would find out soon enough. I made myself a cup of tea and then walked to class.

Once we had all assembled in the classroom, Gordon pulled out a stack of what looked like A4 cardstock. 'Okay, I have your NLP Practitioner certificates here with me, and I will be presenting them to everyone. The first person I am calling up got 50 out of 50, and that is Oliver.'

My jaw dropped. I was speechless.

'Come on up, Oliver', said Gordon. 'Really good work.'

I walked up to the front of the class, and Gordon shook my hand. One of my fellow students had brought her camera to document the ceremony, and she took my picture as Gordon presented me with my certificate. It was a bittersweet moment when we all received our certificates and went our separate ways, concluding our NLP strategic coaching course. As everyone began to leave, I booked my flights for the following month to attend my NLP master practitioner course in Sydney.

If you feel stuck and you're unsure of what you want to do in life, be gentle with yourself and give yourself time to explore. You might not identify your purpose straight away. Sometimes, it may take an event or a peak experience to trigger that realisation. When you allow yourself to dive into the experience, especially with people you trust, it will give you the key to unlock your true passion.

CHAPTER
12

WALKING MY TALK

When you have discovered your purpose and found something that is your true calling, it is up to you to walk the talk and develop an action plan. It will take time and require effort on your part, so it is important to enjoy the journey along the way. When you overcome the obstacles in your path and finally turn your dreams into a reality, you will see that all the hard work and sacrifices have been worth it.

After celebrating my achievement in receiving 100% in my NLP strategic coaching assessment, I soon began to prepare for my upcoming NLP master practitioner course. I booked an Airbnb in Sydney, and before I knew it, I was once again sitting in a classroom with Gordon Young at the helm.

'Today, we are focussing on untangling the Gordian Knot', said Gordon. 'That means, we are seeking to find a simple answer to a seemingly intractable problem. I'm looking for a volunteer for this next exercise. Who has a specific issue that I can work on? It is coming from over here.' He waived his hand towards the part of the room where I was seated.

'I-I will go', I stammered. 'I do tend to get worried easily', I replied.

'Hmm, that is something that I am picking up', said Gordon. 'I'm happy to go with that. Come on up, Oliver. Now what do you tend to worry about?'

I approached Gordon and sat in a chair beside him. 'Mostly, I'm worried about what others may think of me. I know I'm different to others.'

'And what makes you think that you're different?' asked Gordon.

'Well, I haven't been known as the most social person', I said, shaking my head. 'Mainly because I was born with Severe Language Disorder. I started speaking several years later than I should have. I was about four years old, in fact.'

'Oliver, I'm going to say something to you. I am not being dismissive. I want you to listen to my words. Ready?'

I nodded.

Gordon looked me straight in the eyes. Then he said, 'Oliver, I don't think that a lot of people can tell that you have struggled in this way. I want you to let that sink in. I think for most people, you are a great bloke, and that's all that matters. You have overcome many things in your life. *You* see the effects of your language delay. But we don't. We see a kind, caring man. We see a man who is learning to be kind and caring to himself. We see you, and we accept you for who you are. We are all different in our own way, and that is okay. For you to open up about your unique differences is incredibly strong.'

'I used to be ashamed of my language delay', I admitted. 'Now, I'm not as afraid of opening up about it. In a way, it makes me who I am. I guess I'm still just worried that other people will judge me. I tend to get the feeling that others may not like me because of who I am.'

'Okay, let me ask you, how can you determine for absolute certainty what other people are thinking about you?' asked Gordon.

I opened my mouth and then closed it. I shrugged my shoulders.

'I'm going to suggest that you don't know what to say because nobody can determine for certain what another person is thinking about, positive or negative', said Gordon. 'Even if you ask them directly, they might not tell the truth. So, I'm going to suggest a course of action. Don't engage in a worry loop about what may be going on in other people's minds.'

'I don't know what you mean', I said, shaking my head.

'Okay. Let's do an exercise. I'm going to ask you to go outside the room', said Gordon. 'When you're out in the hall, the rest of the class is going to talk.

Then we'll invite you back in.'

'Okay...' I said slowly.

'Very good. Now, go outside. We'll call you back in a bit.' He nodded to Brigitte, the career advisor, who was assisting on the course.

I nodded and reluctantly left the room. I passed several anxious minutes as I waited outside the classroom door.

'Okay, Oliver, we're ready for you now', called Brigitte from inside the room.

As I walked back into the classroom, Gordon said, 'Welcome back, Oliver. Now, I'd like to ask you, out of 10, how strong is your feeling of being worried what the others here think of you?'

'I'm sitting at around an 8', I replied, staring at my shoes.

'Okay, I can see that you are looking down, but I have a feeling that your fear is right in front of you. Now look at me', said Gordon, locking eyes with me. 'What if I took the feeling and tossed it up above you? Would that help?' Gordon moved his arm towards the ceiling.

'That does make a bit of a difference', I replied. 'My fear isn't as intense now.'

'Okay, what if I took the feeling of fear and threw it out the window?' asked Gordon. He made a grabbing motion with his hand and flung the invisible ball of feeling towards a large window on the other side of the room.

'That has made more of a difference', I said. 'It's like the feeling isn't right up in my face anymore.'

WE ARE ALL DIFFERENT IN OUR OWN WAY, AND THAT IS OKAY. FOR YOU TO OPEN UP ABOUT YOUR UNIQUE DIFFERENCES IS INCREDIBLY STRONG.'

'That's right', said Gordon. 'When you are dealing with a feeling, especially a feeling that comes from a limiting belief, it's best to move it further away from you. Make it small and distant, and imagine it in black and white. The less vivid you make it, the less likely it is to keep cycling around and around in your head on a loop. When you interrupt a pattern, it loses its ability to control you.'

I nodded. 'Wow. Yeah, the feeling is getting even less powerful now.'

'On a scale of 10, where is it now?' asked Gordon.

'It's at a 1 or a 2', I said.

'Good', nodded Gordon. 'Now, how do you feel about what others in this room think of you?'

'What others think of me is not relevant to me anymore', I said, a smile spreading slowly across my face. 'Wow. That's pretty incredible.'

'That's good', said Gordon. 'I'm going to let you in on a secret. When you were out of the room just now, the class and I talked about the weather today. We didn't even mention you.'

'Oh!' I exclaimed. 'So, my fear of what the people in class were saying about me...wasn't even real?'

'That's right', nodded Gordon. 'Our worries are just thoughts that we put in our heads. They're often not based in the reality of what is happening. Now, I'm going to ask you a question, and I want your immediate answer. Oliver, why would I want to get to know you?'

'Uh, well', I stammered. 'I'm someone who wants to get to know other people. I take an interest in others.'

'Okay. And...? What else?' asked Gordon.

'I'm also a person who takes action', I said. 'If I have a goal or a vision, I not only plan how to do it, I take active steps to achieve it.'

'Yes. I believe that about you', said Gordon. 'I've seen the evidence. One of the things that I have learnt about you is that you have lost a significant amount of weight over the last year. You have also made huge progress since you began the NLP course. Remember last time? What was your limiting belief?'

'I believed that I could never be loved', I said.

'And what do you say to someone who tells you, "Oliver, you can never be loved"?'

'I say, "You're wrong. I *can* be loved".'

'Good. And what do you say to your own inner voice when you say to yourself, "I can never be loved"?'

'I remind myself, "I *can* be loved. I *deserve* to be loved". I say, "I'm *not afraid* of being loved anymore". That's one of my biggest obstacles. I'm overcoming my fear of rejection.'

'Thank you, Oliver', said Gordon. 'It takes a lot of courage for someone to do what you just did.'

I went back to my Airbnb that evening with a lot of thoughts swimming around in my head. I felt like I was on the verge of another breakthrough. The next morning was the final day of training. If I passed, I would receive my NLP master practitioner certification. I went to sleep early and woke with the dawn the next morning. I wanted to give myself enough time to mentally and emotionally prepare myself to take the next steps into my future.

As I walked into the classroom, Gordon was standing inside the doorway, handing out long, wooden boards to each of the trainees. I took a board and raised my eyebrows. Gordon gave me a mischievous smile.

'You'll see soon', he said in answer to my unstated question.

As soon as the class had assembled, Gordon told us, 'I've given each of you a board. I want you to take out a pen and write on either side of your board. On one side, I want you to write what you want to improve. On the other side, I want you to write what is holding you back.'

I took out a pen and considered what I wanted to write. What were my goals? And what was holding me back? After a few minutes, it came to me. My pen began to move quickly across the board as I jotted down the words that were coming from my heart.

Gordon gave the class about fifteen minutes to complete writing.

'Okay, so as some of you may have guessed, today we will be breaking boards.'

There was a groan, a few gasps, and several squeals of excitement. I looked down at my board. It seemed quite solid. How on earth was I going to break it? It seemed impossible. 'Well, I suppose if any injuries occur, we won't have to worry too much as the RPA is right next door', I said.

Gordon let out a deep belly laugh. 'Yep, we've thought of everything.'

Gordon placed two large bricks on the ground, and then he gestured for us to gather up. We formed a tight circle around the bricks like players preparing for a football match.

'Now, the key is to have your left knee up if you're righthanded', explained Gordon. 'Hold your opposite hand on the brick supporting the board and use your full force. I'm going to show you that you can do this. You're only going to break one board, but I'm going to demonstrate with two.'

Gordon picked up two boards, stacking them one on top of the other, and placed them over the bricks. He raised his right arm up and came down on the boards with the full force of his strength. The boards split evenly in two.

'Now, we'll get the Melbourne guys to go first as I know that you have flights to catch', he said.

I was one of the first to volunteer. I looked at my board before kneeling down to place it on the edge of the two bricks. I read the words I had written on either side, representing my goals and obstacles.

I had written four goals:

1. Being able to build rapport with someone I haven't met without having to be introduced by others.
2. Progressing in my coaching education to become a certified personal fitness trainer.
3. Improving my social skills and my people-reading abilities.
4. Building up the confidence to be in a successful relationship.

I turned the board over and looked at the other side. Staring back at me were the obstacles that had been holding me back for so many years:

1. Fear of rejection.
2. Procrastination and making excuses.
3. Lack of boundaries.
4. Lack of confidence.

I decided to keep my obstacles face up, allowing myself to have a tangible feeling of breaking through these barriers. I bent down to lay my board across the bricks. Then I kneeled on my right knee, steadying myself by placing my left foot on the ground. I secured my left hand on the edge of the brick, and I positioned my right hand over the board.

'Lean right over the top of it', said Gordon as I began raising my right hand.

I used my full force and broke through the board on the first attempt. That was the moment that my true breakthrough happened. It was a metaphor made real. I felt my obstacles fall away as my goals came into focus, just ahead of me on my path. I knew I could accomplish anything I set my mind and heart to achieving.

A month later, I returned to Sydney to qualify as an NLP facilitator. My final exam was to give a presentation about my journey to becoming a coach. I worked on my speech for several days, writing and rewriting it. Finally, it was time to present it to the class. On the morning of my speech, I stood up in front of my fellow coaches-to-be, preparing myself to take the next big step in my life. I took a deep breath, and then I began.

'Hi everyone, my name is Oliver, and I am a health and wellness coach. My passion is helping others to achieve their goals and live a happier and healthier life. I would like to begin by asking if you've ever had a moment where you realised that you needed to make a change?' I looked around the room and saw several heads nodding in agreement. 'I'm sure we all have. Today, I will tell you about a time that I reached an impasse in my life.'

I took a deep breath and steadied myself, silently praying for the courage to share my whole story. 'My life went downhill when I was quite young, due to the constant bullying I received in school. I was clinically depressed, and I contemplated suicide. I decided to seek help, and I got some temporary relief from the pain, but it didn't last for long. Soon, I stopped caring about what I was eating, and I didn't really look after my health. Then, my world turned upside down when my mother was diagnosed with ovarian cancer.'

I paused, fighting back tears. *'Courage, Oliver'*, I thought to myself. After a moment, I took another deep breath, and I forged ahead.

'I was so scared and so depressed', I said, my voice shaking. 'My life was spiralling out of control. I gained 30kg. I reached a point where I just wanted to give up on life. That's when a friend sent me an invitation to a workplace weight loss competition. I was going to give it a pass, but then something inside of me told me that I should do it, even though I was sure I would just give up in three months. Deep down, I knew that enough was enough. I was the only one who could turn my life around, and this time, I was determined to do it.'

> 'OUR WORRIES ARE JUST THOUGHTS THAT WE PUT IN OUR HEADS. THEY'RE OFTEN NOT BASED IN THE REALITY OF WHAT IS HAPPENING.

I looked up at the audience. My classmates were hanging on my every word. It was so quiet that I could have heard a pin drop.

'Even though I initially lacked faith in myself, I committed to making a change. I joined a gym and started exercising five days a week. In a few months, I started seeing results. I lost 28kg in just under a year. My life coach encouraged me to post my journey to social media, publicly sharing the results I'd been achieving in private. This allowed me to lead by example and influence others to change their lives as well.

'Earlier this year, I received a personal invitation to my life coach's retreat in Bali. Little did I know it would change my life. I experienced a profound personal transformation. I released the baggage of fourteen years' worth of negative emotions. At the end of the retreat, I had an epiphany. I knew with complete clarity that it is my life's purpose to become a coach. It is my calling to help others achieve what I have accomplished.

'Recently, I've had another realisation. I want to write a book. As a child, I didn't talk until I was four. My speech therapist diagnosed me with Severe Language Disorder. When I was young, none of my doctors or teachers thought I would ever make it this far in life. By writing a book, I will show the world that you can accomplish anything you set your mind to if you are willing to put in the time, effort, and dedication.

'There's another reason I want to write a book. As a coach, I can help so many more people through the printed word than I can in a one-on-one session. What if I were to show thousands of people how to apply the same simple lifestyle changes that transformed my life? Just imagine the impact that it would have! I now realise that it is my duty to share my story with the world. I've walked my talk to success, and I know that my story will help other people achieve the success that they deserve. Thank you.'

At the end of my speech, my classmates started applauding. Gordon walked over to me, a broad grin on his face. He shook my hand and presented me with my facilitator certificate and my full diploma in NLP Leadership and Coaching. As I stood in front of the class, holding my diploma, I felt immense gratitude for all the struggles and triumphs that had led me to this achievement. It was one of the proudest moments of my life. I had realised my dream of turning my purpose into a reality.

When you commit to fulfilling your purpose, you will have an experience of certainty and direction that will lead you to your life's destination. Think of what actions you need to take that will bring you closer to your goals. Know that there will be obstacles along the way as achieving success is never meant to be an easy path. Everyone has the right to be successful in life, and you do too. Once you turn your purpose into a reality, that's when the true journey begins.

ABOUT THE AUTHOR

Oliver Braykovich is a Master Practitioner of Neuro-Linguistic Programming. He holds a Diploma of NLP, Leadership & Coaching from the Institute of Applied Psychology in Sydney. He is passionate about helping others overcome the obstacles they face in life. This passion stems from personal experience. He was born with Severe Language Disorder, which affected his speech and learning in school. He struggled with his mental and physical health for many years until a workplace weight loss challenge set him on a path of personal transformation. He lost nearly 30kg in a year's time and overcame severe depression and social anxiety. Over the course of that year, he learnt an important lesson about personal growth: when you fully commit to changing your life, the world around you will assist you in your journey. This experience inspired him to become a coach to help other people overcome their own mental and physical health challenges. In Walking My Talk to Success, his goal is to inspire others to level up in their own life and become the best version of themselves.